Social Economics
for the 1970's

Eveline M. Burns
Robert J. Lampman
Garth L. Mangum
Sar A. Levitan
Gerard Piel
Herman M. Somers

Programs for Social
Security, Health
and Manpower

George F. Rohrlich
Editor

Foreword by
Alvin H. Hansen

Social Economics
for the 1970's

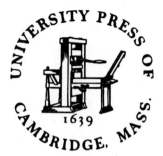

UNIVERSITY PRESS OF
CAMBRIDGE, MASS.
1639

The Dunellen Company, Inc., New York

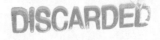

To the memory

of

R. T. R. and E. R.

Foreword

When Professor Rohrlich asked me to write a brief foreword for this volume on social economics for the 1970's, I wondered what one could say in a few paragraphs on so vast a subject. I concluded that perhaps I could best point a finger at the directions that the American economy may reasonably be expected to take and state in a few sentences (necessarily dogmatic in view of the brevity) my views with respect to these developments.

There is today virtually universal agreement—perhaps this in itself should make one skeptical—that the economy will be operating under conditions of excess aggregate demand generated primarily by ever-growing governmental expenditures and strongly reenforced by rapid technological progress.

This poses a problem precisely the opposite of that confronting us in the 1930's. Instead of widespread mass unemployment, we shall be confronted with the problem of saturating the supply of labor to the structure of demand (training of workers, relocation, etc.); and from the standpoint of equilibrium, the problem will be how to adjust aggregate demand to potential aggregate supply without causing an unacceptable degree of inflation.

Fiscal and monetary policy will be stepping on and braking the accelerator. This will be the economist's primary job. But, of course, he may in his spare moments (if any), as indeed he has always done, devote himself to social philosophy—to the burning problems of social priorities: What is it all for? Why growth and equilibrium? What are the ultimate values? As your editor suggests, I have myself not altogether neglected these matters in my own writings. In this Foreword, however, I shall limit myself to what we might call economic mechanics.

If aggregate demand (which all modern governments must massively support) proves to be excessive in relation to potential aggregate supply, then the engineering problem of restraint becomes, for the economist, paramount. Let me here briefly indicate alternative methods for achieving equilibrium.

History shows us that economic equilibrium is not a matter of smoothly adjusting to "lapses from full employment." The economy has always proceeded by fits and starts due particularly to unforeseen events. It is the unexpected earthquake that upsets smooth and happy sailing. And there is no evidence that economic earthquakes are a thing of the past. Consider the year 1966. The gap between actual and potential output had (though somewhat

haltingly) been closing. The long-looked-for 4 per cent unemployment rate
had at long last been reached. A projected curve showed actual growth riding
smoothly on the back of the potential growth curve.

Then came the explosion. The dynamite had already been placed in 1965.
All bets were off. Huge bulges of aggregate demand, fed by a big jump in
military expenditures and reenforced by private fixed investment, swept the
economy along the road ahead. No computer could foresee what would
happen.

The drivers at the wheel were offered a choice of three ways to put on the
brakes: (1) taxation, (2) monetary policy—money supply and interest
rates—and (3) controls.

Having caught the vision of a happy land overflowing with milk and
honey—the 1964 tax reduction had raised hopes of further reductions—the
Congress and the public were in no mood for a contracylclical fiscal policy.
And so, not until 1968 did we get even a moderate tax surcharge. Tax brakes
being applied belatedly and sparingly, the easy and popular alternative was
monetary policy. Two things seem to me to be conclusive as one takes a hard
look at this experiment: (a) as an overall check on aggregate demand, it just
did not do the job; (b) instead of reestablishing equilibrium, it created serious
distortions and discriminatioas in the economy.

Taking the second point first, so much has been written about the
seriously discriminating impact of the restrictive monetary policy on housing
and on state and local government bond issues that I need only mention it
here. With respect to the first point, why did monetary restraint not act
effectively to check aggregate demand before inflation got well on its way?

To this there are several answers. When the increase in the money supply is
restricted in relation to an upsurge in aggregate demand, the difference is
partly made up by an increase in velocity. Hard pressed by a high rate of
interest, business concerns released a part of their own cash balances for
active investment. Moreover, they obtained the money needed for expansion
partly by tapping the growing internal flow of funds. Corporate profits after
taxes and dividends plus capital consumption allowances increased from
$63.1 billion in 1964 to $75.4 billion in 1969. Bank loans to business
increased from $167.7 billion in 1964 to $276.2 billion in 1969. This was
made possible, despite monetary restraint, partly by unloading government
securities and by the sale of negotiable certificates of deposit, partly by
drawing funds away from savings and loan associations and partly by tapping
Euro-dollars. Thus, private investment in plant and equipment kept on rising
at an accelerated rate—rising from $56.8 billion in 1964 to $94 billion in
1969. The ratio of investment in plant and equipment to gross national
product was 9.8 per cent. This equaled the extraordinary rate of 9.7 per cent
in 1956-57.

But why didn't the rapidly rising interest rate restrain the rising volume of fixed capital investment? An adequate answer to this question would involve an examination in depth of the shape of the marginal efficiency of capital schedule—the relation of the volume of investment to the rate of interest.[1] Is the investment-demand schedule interest elastic or interest inelastic? Wicksell and Keynes believed it to be inelastic. Cassel and Fisher (and current monetarists) believed it to be elastic. If it were indeed interest elastic, investment should have been choked off sharply in the period 1966-69. The opposite proved to be the case.

Thus, the conflict between the monetary theorists and the fiscal-policy theorists simmers down pretty much to a difference of opinion with respect to the interest elasticity of investment. If the schedule is interest inelastic, it does little good, from the standpoint of restraint, to raise the interest rate. What is needed is to shift the investment demand schedule to the left by fiscal policy measures.

If, as I believe, monetary policy is both discriminatory and ineffective as an anti-inflationary measure, does this mean that monetary policy is of no account? By no means. Monetary policy should and must play an important role if we are to achieve optimum growth. Growth requires that investment (private and public) must exceed saving (private and public), so that tomorrow's income may exceed today's income. For the long-run pull, the gap must be filled by new money. I am quite prepared to accept Milton Friedman's 4 per cent per annum increase in the money supply, provided he will then allow me a fiscal policy (both short term and long term) adequate to ensure reasonable price stability and full employment.[2] Rather than a fixed 4 per cent rule, however, I should prefer a less rigid rule—a monetary policy that would give us a stable low rate of interest.

But if it proves to be politically impossible, at least in the near future, to offset the expected rapidly growing rate of public expenditures by the appropriate level of taxation, what then? There remain wage and price controls. Yet here, also, there is strong current opposition. The most that I can see over the horizon is a six-month cooling-off period. The giant corporations in the administered price areas (in which a few leaders dominate the field) should be required to delay for six months any proposed price increase. This would enable the government to publicize full data on costs and prices. It would be hoped that full publicity might prove to be a considerable restraining force. Continuous education (with governmental support) with respect to the importance and role of wage-price guide lines should vigorously be resumed.

Looking further ahead, it is wholly utopian to believe that we shall one day at long last establish a Fiscal Policy Board, operating under authority of the President, with power to alter the income tax surcharge (both negatively and positively) together with an investment-tax credit (both negative and positive)—such changes to be subject to Congressional veto within 30 days? "Five-year plans" with respect to public expenditures should be prepared by the Council of Economic Advisers, together with continuous surveys looking toward basic changes and reforms in the overall tax structure.[3]

I fear that even this brief analysis reveals how desperately far we are from having solved the problem of price stability and full employment.[4] The conventional pattern of thinking still fatalistically accepts what is called a moderate level of unemployment, say 4 or 5 per cent. Can this defeatist approach survive in the disturbing social upheaval through which we are currently passing?

A skit of Art Buchwald's (humor with a sting) hits the nail on the head. Art congratulates a newly discharged worker for joining the "elite" group which is making such a "valuable contribution" in the fight against inflation. Presenting his friend with a Certificate of Unemployment, Art assures him that he can be very proud to be among the chosen few drafted to keep the economy from spiraling. Worker: "Gosh, it's beautiful. Wait until my family sees it."

Unemployment is the cruellest form of regressive redistribution of income. It punishes those least able to bear the social cost of achieving price stability. No government would *deliberately* impose this kind of utterly intolerable discrimination. It all happens in the normal operation of the price system!

The Nixon Administration's guaranteed minimum income is on the right track. But it is hopelessly inadequate. A basic annual minimum could, however, be built around a year comprising 2,000 working hours. At the legal minimum hourly wage of $1.60 per hour, this would mean a yearly guaranteed income of $3,200. The figure should be raised whenever the legal minimum hourly wage is increased. This program, I suggest, is the very least that society can do for those who perform the thankless task of easing the pressure of an inflationary boom. Of course, those unemployed workers should be trained and relocated, so that they can compete effectively in a world of changing skills. This revolving labor group would provide a much needed flexibility to a dynamic labor market.

Alvin H. Hansen
Lucius N. Littauer Professor
of Political Economy, Emeritus
Harvard University

Notes

1. Alvin H. Hansen, *Monetary Theory and Fiscal Policy* (New York: McGraw-Hill, 1949), Chapters 4 and 5.

2. By "reasonable price stability," I mean approximate stability of wholesale prices say, possibly, a 1 per cent increase per year. On this basis however, consumer prices could be expected to rise by 2 or 2½ per cent per year, in view of the low level of productivity increases in the services area. It may well be that we shall follow Western Europe and accept a 3.5 per cent increase in consumer prices.

3. A good beginning has been made in the 1970 Economic Report.

4. In February 1970 the New York *Times* reported that the Canadian government has become convinced that the conventional tools for fighting inflation were failing to do the job within political limits.

Preface

Writing about the decade following World War II, Harvard's distinguished political economist Alvin H. Hansen made an appraisal of postwar economic developments in the United States.[1] With obvious professional pride, he noted the years of sustained "almost incredible *output* performance" and our "great advances on the purely economic plane" to which "economists, as a professional group ... contributed in no small measure." At the same time, he was critical of the outcome at large and of the economists' share in it. He pointed to the nation's shortfalls in decent housing and education and to its gadget-ridden but culturally deficient life styles and concluded: "We have learned how to make a living, we have still to learn how to live." Economists, he felt, had been neglectful of their duty in not bespeaking public needs and not devoting more study to social priorities.[2]

In the intervening years, America's economy, as measured by all the indicators in use, has grown further and has achieved the longest unbroken prosperity period on record; unemployment reached the lowest point it ever had, outside of periods of global war; poverty has declined, both proportionally and in absolute numbers. Yet, the socioeconomic dislocations which marred the picture in Hansen's stock-taking are more pronounced and more apparent today than they were then. Following the appearance in 1962 of Michael Harrington's *The Other America,* the once "invisible poor" have become plainly visible, and vocal to boot—what with the bold proclamation of a "War on Poverty" in which those to be helped were to exert "maximum feasible participation." Economists have turned in increasing numbers to studying problems of poverty and possible ways to eradicate it or, at least, to cope with its ill effects. The more we study and experiment, the wider and deeper are the interconnections and ramifications that we discover to be linking together the various disfunctional aspects of our socio-economic fabric.

Concomitantly, the vision of a Great Society that

> rests on abundance and liberty for all, [which] demands an end to poverty and racial injustice ... where every child can find knowledge to enrich his mind and to enlarge his talents ... where the city of man serves ... the desire for beauty and the hunger for community ... where men are more concerned with the quality of their goals than the quantity of their goods,

though no less inspiring today than when President Johnson first raised it before the eyes of the American people,[3] appears ever more awesome and remote. The lesson to be drawn must be, not to abandon its pursuit, but to broaden and intensify our search for tractable causes and for workable solutions that bring optimum leverage to bear at strategic points.

The problem and policy areas to be explored cover a wide range—too wide to encompass within the covers of a slim volume such as the present one. It is easily possible to make different selections of certain key areas, either on grounds that they are most in need of corrective action or because they are the most promising of success, with beneficial spillover effects beyond their own confines, and hence most deserving to be brought to the attention of the reading public and especially those who have a particular concern with public policy. This volume addresses itself to three problem and policy areas of cardinal import: social security, in the broad sense of providing for the essentials in the common contingencies; health care, modes of delivery that give the best assurance of meeting needs; and manpower, the development of earning capacity through skill-training. The major contributors are distinguished authorities in their respective fields, and the discussants, likewise, are long-time students or practitioners. The treatments included in Part 2 attempt to set the stage, i.e., they provide a conceptual or historical overview. Those in Part 3 deal more specifically with existing or proposed programs. These presentations are based on a series of symposia held in 1969 under the auspices of the newly established Institute for Social Economics and Policy Research at Temple University in Philadelphia. Part 1 contains some explanatory remarks as regards the meaning and scope of social economics, a field that, even though it deals with problems many of which are far from new, is only now emerging as a distinct area of economic study and analysis. This and the concluding Part IV were supplied by the editor, who is the Director of the Institute and who acted as chairman for the symposia.

Warm thanks are due to the School of Business Administration of Temple University and, in particular, to Dr. Seymour L. Wolfbein, its dynamic Dean, for the funding and for much other help in the establishment of the Institute and its inaugural program, of which the series of symposia here reported was a part; to Dr. Simon Slavin, Dean of the School of Social Administration, and to Dr. Leroy E. Burney, Vice-President for Health Sciences of Temple University, who took turns with Dean Wolfbein in chairing and moderating the symposia. Thanks are due also to the U.S. Department of Labor for financial support derived from its Manpower Research Institutional Grant to Temple University, and to the administrator of the grant, Dr. Louis T. Harms, Associate Dean, School of Business Administration, for his never-failing encouragement. Last, but by no means least, I wish to acknowledge my debt of gratitude to the staff of the Dunellen Publishing Company for their encouragement and help in getting the manuscript ready for the printer in record time. Most particularly I am indebted to Paule H. Jones, Executive Editor, for her generous help and competent advice.

Notes

1. Hansen, *The American Economy* (New York: McGraw-Hill, 1957).

2. Ibid., pp. 146-150.

3. From President Lyndon B. Johnson's speech on the campus of the University of Michigan at Ann Arbor, May 22, 1964, as quoted in *The Great Society Reader,* edited by M. E. Gettleman and D. Mermelstein (New York: Vintage Books, 1967), p. 16.

Contents

List of Tables and Figures

Tables

Figures

Part 1   Introduction

1

The Challenge of
Social Economics

George F. Rohrlich

Until "free exchange" and "social reform" are both interpreted as governed by one consistent set of laws, they are not interpreted correctly. The crucial task of such a theory is to reveal those causes and consequences of things men do which transcend the scope of free exchange. These create responsibilities which, in turn, the policy of regulation is attempting to enforce. In a broad sense the great task of the theorist of our tremendously dynamic age is to substitute an economics of responsibility for the economics of irresponsible conflict.[1]

John Maurice Clark

In this age of slogans and catchwords, we have become habituated to a wellnigh continuous stream of phrases and expressions—some new, some old with a new twist—that purport to articulate people's needs or wants, and ways to meet them. Their wide range encompasses virtually any aspect of the human condition or aspiration, from a supposed desire for "pucker power" in a mouthwash to the professed need for "relevance" in education through novel forms of—and funding for—more effective community participation in the governance of our educational institutions, as well as wide-open admissions policies by the centers of higher learning. The variety and multiplicity of competing claims upon our national resources to meet such vastly different demands, not to mention the excruciating choices between the alleged needs of national and world security, on the one hand, and the furtherance of domestic wellbeing, on the other, are bewildering to citizens and policy makers alike.

The Limitations of the Market Place and the Need for Broader Horizons

Earlier generations of economists, observing the working of their contemporary economies, were able to sustain a faith in "pre-established harmonies"—as did the Physiocrats—or in the guidance of an "invisible hand"—as did Adam Smith—whereby the pursuit of self-interest by each

I am grateful to my colleague Professor Karl Niebyl for his willingness to read the manuscript of his chapter and for his helpful comments.

individual would mysteriously bring about the reconciliation and maximization of the interests of all.[2]

This soothing, if simplistic, faith has often come under attack, most prominently by political dissidents, those opposed to the capitalist system as such, but also—and increasingly—by school economists, members of the fraternity, whose criticism was motivated by a desire to improve the functioning and the stability of our economic system rather than by a desire to destroy or to replace it. One of the targets of their criticism has been the sovereign and elated role traditionally assigned to the "market place" and to the value judgments that govern it.

One such challenge was raised well over half a century ago by one of America's foremost economists, John Maurice Clark. In his quest for a concept of "Social Value," which he thought "an economist should be prepared to face ... with all its difficulties" he formulated three basic propositions:

> (1) that ... the collective efficiency of private enterprise involves quantities of which actual market prices are not the only measure, and ... some of which command no market price at all ... (2) that measures of value which may be less exact than those of the market are also much more fundamental ...; and (3) that our most fundamental concepts should be independent of institutions of competitive exchange ...[3]

Another distinguished American economist, Alvin H. Hansen, wrote in a similar vein more than a dozen years ago:

> The "market" cannot decide how much we shall spend on schools, on social security, or on national security. We have reached a point in our economic and social evolution where *social-value* judgments, not the market, must control the uses to which we put something like one-fourth of our productive resources. Our economy is no longer wholly a market economy. It is a mixed public-private economy .... Civilized countries mold their people into civilized ways of thinking, guided by values that experience and knowledge have laid down. We don't leave it to the market. We educate. Only in this way can we achieve the great goals of a civilized society.[4]

Of all the critics among American economists of the leave-it-to-the-market concept, none has subjected the promotional, "contrived" character of want creation with regard to material goods that takes place in the private sector of the American economy to a more searching scrutiny or a more scathing indictment than John K. Galbraith.[5] He has charged that private wants have come to depend increasingly on high-pressure advertising; that instead of actual wants resulting in the production of the commodities desired, it is the newly marketed and much advertised commodity that brings forth a desire to own it. Such artifically kindled desires, even if intense and widespread, cannot be said to arise in spontaneous consumer needs. A system thus propelled and catering to created wants can hardly be viewed as responding to needs in any meaningful sense of the term, nor can it be assumed "that [under such conditions] welfare is greater at an all-around higher level of production than at a lower one." On the contrary, there is bound to ensue a "tendency to provide an opulent supply of some things and a niggardly yield of others."[6] Private goods and services (bought in the market place) tend to fall in the former category; those available for social consumption (i.e., by the use of a public facility or service) tend to fall in the latter ("Theory of Social [Un-] Balance").[7]

It would be tempting to apply the same criteria to other areas of human endeavor to see if they are impervious to this reproach. As regards human preferences or wants in the field of politics, for example, does the promotion of a new candidate, or sometimes of a new idea, take forms that are very different from the commercial promotion of a new product? With regard to social movements generally, do not the protagonists of a cause also seek to arouse and play on needs or responses often far from conscious and concrete, sometimes perhaps only dormant before being articulated and played up? Moreover, does the allocation of a growing share of the national product to the public sector necessarily further social consumption of the kind Galbraith favors? Cannot high-powered lobbies significantly influence the formulation of our supposed public wants and needs as much as our private ones are ever manipulated?[8] Last, can all changes in private demand be understood in like manner? To use a drastic example, could Galbraith's model explain the dramatic rise in the consumption of mind-distorting drugs over the last decade or so? Can that "demand" be interpreted simply as a "dependence effect", i.e., as the induced result of high-pressure salesmanship—unadvertised, to be sure, but supported by an efficient distribution and marketing system of illicit, yet well organized, purveyors? It does not seem plausible. Even a more broadly conceived demonstration effect could not, by itself, furnish enough of an explanation. The individual motivations and social forces at work are, no doubt, far more complex.

Regardless, however, of the exhaustiveness or universal applicability of Galbraith's thesis as to why it is that the direction of our economic pursuits and the framework and gauges commonly used to evaluate our economic performance are so one-sided, the correctness of his observation—and similar observations of the other critics—that this *is* the case is incontrovertible. Alongside the ever-growing private wealth, there are clearly, and for all to see, the acute problems that confront our system of public education, the ominous shortcomings in personal and environmental health care, the decay that engulfs a growing portion of our housing stock, the inadequacy of urban transportation, and many others. Less obvious to some, but not less real, are the scars which these disfunctional aspects of our national economy have left on important segments of the population by reason of unmet needs, gaps in acculturation, squalor, and the waste of human potential—notably, but by no means exclusively, among minority members, and engulfing significant numbers of children and youths. The latest, but perhaps not the ultimate, fall-out products of massive proportions are civic discontent, mutual fear and alienation, and various more severe forms of social or socially induced pathology.

Incomplete and Deceptive Measures of Progress and the Need for Complementary Gauges

Some conceptual and methodological failings associated with this lopsidedness were highlighted, fairly recently and rather persuasively, in the Report of the National Commission on Technology, Automation, and Economic Progress.[9] Referring to the limitations of our national economic progress, the Commission pointed out that "GNP measures only market transactions"; that it "does not adequately reflect . . . side effects in the form of social costs and benefits"; and that the national aggregates "tell us little about pockets of poverty, depressed communities, sick industries, or disadvantaged social groups."[10]

The Commission judged that these macroeconomic measures developed in the 1930's in response to what was thought to be necessary information at the time (and still is, to be sure) and since then collected by the government, "shaped in considerable measure the subsequent direction of economic theory and practice." Among the distortions of our present gauges of economic growth, the Commission mentioned, for example, the "additive" nature of our GNP accounting, which lends it a deceptive growth bias in the following manner: ". . . when a factory is built, the new construction and the new payrolls are an addition to GNP." If at the same time the factory pollutes a stream, our present GNP measures will not record this unless and until the factory

> builds a filtration plant to divert the wastes [in which case] these expenditures, too, become an addition to GNP. In the financial sense, more money has been spent in the economy. But the gross addition simply masks an "offset cost," not a contribution to economic progress.[11]

Conversely, a downward bias in estimating the value of goods and services produced flows from the noninclusion, with certain exceptions, of those unpaid. As a result, one might point to the fact—as an example of other paradoxical consequences—that parental neglect necessitating that a child be entrusted to foster care is reflected in our present aggregative accounting as a net addition to the national product.

The thought that concepts and measures are bound to influence the definition of subject matter, as well as analytic approaches and the focus for action, prompted the Commission to top its findings in this area with a set of recommendations clearly aimed at bringing about through new concepts and measures what it judged to be a much-needed compensatory point of view. Specifically, it called for the establishment of a

> system of social accounts . . . [to] give us a broader and more balanced reckoning of the meaning of social and economic progress and . . . move us toward measurement of the utilization of human resources in our society in four areas:
> 1. The measurement of social costs and net returns of economic innovation;
> 2. The measurement of social ills (e.g., crime, family disruption);
> 3. The creation of performance budgets in areas of defined social needs (e.g., housing, education);
> 4. Indicators of economic opportunity and social mobility.

"Eventually", the Commission hoped,

> this might provide a "balance sheet" which could be useful in clarifying policy choices. It would allow us to record not only the gains of economic and social change but the costs as well, and to see how these costs are distributed and borne.[12]

In March 1966, the very next month after the Commission's report was published, President Johnson directed the Secretary of Health, Education and Welfare "to search for ways to improve the Nation's ability to chart its social progress."[13] Secretary John W. Gardner appointed a panel of social scientists from within, as well as outside, the government to advise on the development of "social indicators" to measure social change (in obvious analogy to the "economic indicators" long familiar as measures of economic change) and to help with the possible preparation of a social report comparable to the Economic Report rendered annually by the President's Council of Economic Advisers. In the beginning of 1969, the Department submitted to the President the product of its own and the advisory panel's labors, in the form of a set of preliminary findings and recommendations, titled *Toward a Social Report.*[14]

The Report reviewed currently available statistics and gauges of progress in seven important areas of social well-being: health and illness; social mobility; physical environment; income and poverty; public order and safety; learning; science, and art; and participation and alienation. A "social indicator," as the term is used in the Report, was defined therein as

> a statistic of direct normative interest which facilitates concise, comprehensive and balanced judgment about the condition of major aspects of a society . . . a different measure of welfare . . . subject to the interpretation that, if it changes in the "right" direction, while other things remain equal, things have gotten better, or people are "better off".[15]

Mere program caseloads or expenditures normally do not constitute such indicators, since they do not reveal unequivocally or even inferentially whether ground was gained or lost in the above sense. As an example of a true indicator, the Report cited an index of "healthy life expectancy," i.e., life expectancy free of bed-disability and institutionalization. In most of the areas surveyed, despite a plethora of relevant information on the incidence of various syndromes, as well as plentiful operational data derived from ongoing programs, there was found to be a dearth of true indicators.

The development of true social indicators in each of the major social policy areas, the Commission thought, should add up to "a balanced, organized and concise set of measures of the condition of our society" that would yield "the information needed to identify emerging problems and to make knowledgeable decisions about national priorities." A logical next step would be to produce comparative cost-benefit information relative to alternative programs at various levels of funding. The ultimate objective was to "integrate our social indicators into policy accounts which would allow us to estimate the changes in a social indicator that could be expected to result from alternative levels of expenditure on relevant public programs."[16]

Tha nature of this agenda reinforces the case for a value system that transcends the market economy to which reference was made earlier. In fact, both propositions complement each other: Any authentic indicators of social progress or, for that matter, economic progress redefined (with greater emphasis on qualitative characteristics, even within the market economy, as well as beyond it) would appear to presuppose consistent and coherent theories of value that can provide a solid frame of reference. For it seems impossible to ascertain, let alone measure, progress of any kind, unless one knows where he desires to go. This, in turn, implies a reasoned answer to the question why he wants to get there. Then, of course, in order to know whether we are in fact getting nearer our goals, we need to develop more telling gauges than we now have.

The Emerging Field of Social Economics

From what has been said, it is apparent that the unexplored or at least underexplored dimension of the traditional framework of economic analysis and policy research involves conditions and consequences of man's economic activities and economic satisfactions that either impinge upon or fall squarely within other realms of man's social existence. Among the phenomena in dire need of being better understood and more fully taken into account are the connecting links and the mutual impacts between the purely economic and other, partly contiguous and partly, perhaps, even more remote phases of our existence.

Among the many penetrating and discerning formulations of which Galbraith has shown himself a master, one of deceptive simplicity is a restatement of the traditional definition of the "most urgent requirements of man." To the three most commonly enumerated, viz., food, clothing and shelter, Galbraith adds a fourth: "an orderly environment in which the first three might be provided."[17] It is this fourth requirement—no less urgent than any one of the others—that has commonly been treated lightly, whenever it has not been overlooked altogether. Just how crucial its importance, not only historically, "in the world into which economics was born" (as Galbraith put it) but, if anything, even more in the world that surrounds us today, may become more evident, perhaps, by adding to the last three words, "might be provided," the further condition, "and can be enjoyed." If in the traditional economic setting this fourth condition was a *sine qua non* for the success of the self-reliant individual, the much-vaunted self-made man—through a whole host of social institutions, partly permissive, partly protective, enabling, developmental, supportive—it not only continues to serve this function in the vastly more complex economy of our own day but has become an essential prerequisite for a reasonably smooth functioning of the market economy as a whole.

Astonishingly little attention was paid by a long line of economists to this conditioning or qualifying role of the environment (in more senses than one) either in relation to the satisfaction of human needs or wants, i.e., from the consumer's point of view, or in conjunction with the factors of production, i.e., from the producer's point of view. In the latter respect, perhaps no single cause is more to be credited with alerting us to the "fourth condition's" cardinal importance than our preoccupation, in the last quarter of a century, with the problems of economic development in the economically underdeveloped areas of the world. Not only has our early experience in attempting to cope with the problems of this awesome task more fully opened our eyes to the crucial role of a material infrastructure; it has caused us to assign a far greater importance than it had occupied with generations of economists to the challenge and promise of investment in man or, better, human development. From the vantage point of the consumer's interest, on the other hand, a comparable insight, slower to come by but rapidly advancing at present, has just been gained over the past several years. Its starting point, as well as the continuing leverage that has endowed it with growing momentum, has been the dramatic deterioration of the conditions of urban living. It has received further strong impetus from a growing awareness of the impact of mass production and consumption under conditions of a technologically far-advanced state of the arts on the ecology of our planet.[18] The directions in which this understanding needs to be broadened and

deepened and the ways in which the knowledge gained can be applied to
economic analysis and policy shall be explored in the concluding section of
this essay. To do this must be a central concern of social economics in the
years to come.

But what is social economics? Is it a brand of theoretical or of applied
economics or both? Is there justification for setting it apart as a subdiscipline,
either by reason of differences in approach and methods used or because of
its special subject matter and concerns? Or is it merely another term in the
forever lengthening list of clever plays on words and the suggestive use of
semantics referred to at the outset?

The designation "social economics" itself is, perhaps, more familiar in
Great Britain than in this country.[19] One in the series of the Cambridge
Economic Handbooks deals with this subject and is thus titled.[20] In an initial
chapter, "The Scope and Meaning of Social Economics," an attempt is made
to define the subject matter. Referring to Alfred Marshall's views on the
frontiers of economics generally, to the effect that "there is a large debatable
ground in which economic considerations are of considerable but not
dominant importance; and each economist may reasonably decide for himself
how far he will extend his labours over that ground,"[21] the author, Walter
Hagenbuch, deems it "quite sufficient to say that social economics is
whatever social economists study, and to point to the chapter headings of this
book". He cautions that "the social economist should realize that his study is
essentially a frontier activity, and that in pursuing it he may often cross and
recross the boundary of neighboring social sciences . . ."[22] The chapter
headings referred to are "Population," "Housing," "Working Conditions,"
"Poverty," and, comprising several chapters, "Voluntary and Public Social
Services," including specifically "National Insurance and Assistance." The
distribution of incomes, and education were left out, according to the
author's preface, for no other reason than lack of space. By way of a
functional definition, Hagenbuch sums up the social economist's concern and
activity in a fourfold manner:

(1) as a branch of applied economics: the application of economic
theory to social problems;
(2) as a branch of applied statistics: the numerical measurement of the
extent and constitution of social problems;
(3) as the study of the social causes of economic behavior, which might
be called economic ecology;
(4) as the study of the social consequences of economic behavior,
which some would call welfare economics.[23]

Hagenbuch's conceptual framework can serve as a suitable point of departure
for further examination. Certain modifications will suggest themselves in the
course of this inquiry.

Social Economics as a Branch of Applied Economics

There can be no doubt that certain areas of social need have grown to such proportions and have attained such predominant importance within the national economy and social fabric as to call for the attention of social scientists of many disciplines. The interest and concern of economists, in particular, is amply warranted by the large and increasing share of national product represented by private and public expenditures in these areas that are devoted to bringing forth the goods and services necessary to meet market demand and such nonmarket needs as are deemed compelling enough to be defrayed from tax revenues and other compulsory levies.

The wide scope and the intricacies of subject matter of these several areas call for specialized knowledge going beyond the common tools of the economic generalist. Robert J. Lampman, in a thoughtful and comprehensive review article referred to the economics of health, education, and welfare as lying "inside the methodological frame of general economics," yet constituting an emerging subdiscipline—and possibly a future "school"—with descriptive, normative, and particularly predictive tasks and attributes of its own, as well as with its particular contribution to finding the best answers to the more general aggregative, allocative and distributive questions.[24] Several good examples of the poignant significance and the mutual relevance of different types of expertise and outlook contributed by economists and other specialists, and the interrelationship between the last-mentioned "leading questions of economics" and the aforementioned "moods of inquiry" (to use Lampman's terminology) can be found in Parts 2 and 3 of this book. One of these reveals itself in the positions taken by some of the contributors on the problems of health services delivery. Addressing themselves to the issues bearing on (1) the proper means of expanding health services (aggregative question); (2) what services to provide in greater quantity and in what manner (allocative question); and (3) how to improve their delivery (distributive question), several of these experts come up with their considered judgment, surprising to some, no doubt, that the mere infusion of more money (leaving other things unchanged) might make matters worse, rather than better.

There appears to be no cogent reason why the foregoing observations with regard to the fields of health, education, and welfare might not be extended just as aptly to other fields of applied economics with particularly strong social overtones that have a reasonably clear separate identity, such as social security and manpower development (which Lampman encompassed under his broadly defined categories of "welfare" and "education," respectively), housing, and even certain aspects of transportation. It may suffice to identify as one facet of the emerging subdiscipline the development and application of

suitable analytic concepts and techniques that lend themselves to being used
to good advantage in the subject areas referred to without attempting, at the
present juncture, to give an exhaustive enumeration.

A strong case can be made for the further proposition that some of the
more general concepts and constructs used in economics are in need of
broadening and adaptation specifically in connection with this task. Again, J.
M. Clark's early explorations contain interesting precedents along such lines
and have established targets which, to this day, have not been fulfilled.

Perhaps most striking among the precedents is Clark's extension, after
exhaustive studies of the economics of overhead costs in different sectors of
the economy, of the concept of overhead costs to labor, i.e., to the human
factor in production. This extension of a familiar concept into an until then
untried field of application led to fruitful new insights. It set us on the path
of uncovering the numerous "features of the human cost of labor
corresponding to some of the particular phases of overhead costs in
connection with large fixed capital."[25] This, in turn, may have opened up
vistas for a rethinking of the proper distribution of the burden of maintaining
(or restoring) the laborer's ability to work and, as a direct result thereof,
paved the way for important statutory reforms, notably in the areas of work
injury and unemployment compensation, and other types of social legislation.
The current drives for guaranteed annual wages and for guaranteed minimum
incomes may be seen as latter-day emanations of this then new trend of
thought.

Among Clark's targets that have remained unfulfilled to this day is the
development of more adequate theoretical foundations of certain key
concepts. Foremost among these—which it was his hope that economists
would overcome—is what he called the insulated position of the theory of
value and distribution. He was groping for

> a concept of economic value and valuation with reference to society as
> a whole, independent of market valuations and capable of scientific
> application to concrete cases ... an intellectual instrument that will
> pierce the insulation and establish a connection with the ideas that are
> making things happen.[26]

To evolve the consistent theory which Clark postulated must surely be high
on the agenda of the emerging—or, in view of Clark's own pioneering work,
re-emerging—subdiscipline of social economics. Clark himself, essayed various
different approaches in attempting to define the subject matter more
precisely and devise analytical tools to explore it. "The world is full of unpaid
costs and unappropriated services" he wrote, giving as examples of unpaid
costs "robbing the neighbors of their light and air, obstructing the streets,
fouling streams, increasing or destroying the beauty of the landscape or the
business character of the neighborhood ..." And with reference to

unappropriated services he spoke of ideas and inventions, growth-promoting institutions and favorable environments conducive to individual success—all of which fall short of being "fully appropriable rights," and many of which are altogether "inappropriable," either by their very nature (as social goods—e.g., public sanitation) or because society has chosen not—or not yet—to grant proprietary rights concerning them in full or in part.[27] More remains to be said on this, under a different heading, below.

Social Economics as a Staging Area for Social Accounting

Almost imperceptibily, a second facet of the subdiscipline of social economics, and another important segment of its agenda, has come to the fore: the task of tracing causal relationships and, insofar as possible, quantitative as well as qualitative concatenations between economic activities and social outcomes, i.e., their impact on prevailing social conditions. The task is a composite one. It requires, first of all, the development of conceptual specifications and technical measurements for a fuller stock-taking of all the outputs flowing from defined economic inputs. This means (a) taking account of the known results not heretofore included in our economic calculus, and (b) exploring such further results as have heretofore escaped our attention, either because they fall through the particular conceptual grid economists have been using or because they are altogṣther outside the purview of the field of economics, at least as now defined. The second, and further, task is, then, to identify and relate, if possible in terms of a functional relationship, magnitudes of economic inputs of various kinds to social outcomes, i.e., to ensuing changes in social conditions. The achievement of this objective would correspond to what the National Commission and the subsequent HEW Report referred to as "Performance Budgets" or "Policy Accounts."

The present subsection is intended to deal only with the first-named task. Hagenbuch's "applied statistics" criterion, i.e., "the numerical measurement of the extent and constitution of social problems," describes a part but not all of it. In its place, therefore, the term "social accounting" recommends itself, which is intended to comprise and convey these identification and measurement components, as well as a locational designation within the chain of cause and effect.[28] The hoped-for construction of new gauges of social progress and of a conceptual framework that reflects developments susceptible to being assessed with this end in view lends further meaning and importance to this focus on "social accounting."

The necessary starting point whould appear to be a common-sense critique—from the vantage point of a social accounting—of the "profit (or gain)-and-loss" calculus commonly applied to transactions in the marketplace. In this calculus, as performed by each of the parties involved, i.e., the individual seller or firm and the individual buyer or buying unit (family, household), any consequence of a transaction that does not enter either on the plus or minus side falls, by definition, outside of the valuation process. Thus, a great many consequences elude the valuations of the market place; e.g., the costs of an industrial accident or of industrial waste production enter into the seller's calculus only insofar as they accrue to him, and they fail to enter into it insofar as they are met by others or go—at least in part, or for limited periods of time entirely—unmet. The buyer, similarly, weighs his gain from an exchange in terms of his (and only his) costs, not counting (and seldom caring about) the above-cited or yet other untoward effects, such as resource depletion, that are real enough but the incidence of which is diffused and often unclear.

Popular views of the market as the regulator of values commonly ignore these spillover effects. Even economists have for the longest time paid insufficient attention to them. They have coined a term, "externalities," which has served to identify the phenomenon, and they distinguish two types of these, depending on whether the by-products or side-effects that do not accrue to the firm are benign and, hence, result in gains for others (in which case they are called external economies) or deleterious (in which case they are called external dyseconomies). But in either case, these external, or spillover, effects have been regarded, with the noteworthy exception referred to in the following subsection, as of little or merely occasional importance. For the most part, their existence has been ignored. Only if and when, at long last, an external dyseconomy became too much of a nuisance or burden was remedial action sought from government, either through regulatory action or through legislation (e.g., antipollution ordinances or statutory provisions to pay compensation for death and disability due to occupational diseases). In the meantime, these costs have accrued all along, but they have been met in ways largely unaccounted for, e.g., in the form of a deterioration of the environment or, at any rate, remained unallocated, as in the cost of relief for an occupational injury victim who had become a public charge.

More recently, the frequent presence and importance of such unaccounted-for emanations of economic transactions has become recognized, and ways have been sought of taking them into account in determining the welfare implications of economic output. Concomitantly with and even prior to the study of the subject undertaken by the HEW Panel on Social Indicators, several individual and team efforts were undertaken covering the same ground. These resulted in more comprehensive, scholarly disquisitions on the methodological problems involved, and possible ways of overcoming them.[29] Some explorations reported in these volumes, notably A. W. Sametz's efforts to develop a "welfare-output indicator" and various supplementary indicators of "social welfare and happiness," constitute interesting contributions toward evolving new analytic tools. Sametz looks to a future welfare indicator as revealing "real per capita output per unit of input ... truly net of all costs masquerading as product and gross of nonpriced but real social costs."[30] He views "social cost accounting" as "an essential supplement to the national output accounts (even if the latter are recast ...) for measuring economic progress." He readily admits that such an "output index ... cannot be any more than a partial indicator of social welfare ..."[31]

The attainment of such an aggregate measure would constitute, indeed, a significant forward step. No less and perhaps even more important, however, would be the disaggregation of the findings that led up to it. We need to know the full benefits and the full costs of our economic activities as they affect each of the major areas of human wellbeing. To make this assessment, we need reliable gauges of wellbeing in each of these areas and we need to know how various economic activities, i.e., the production and consumption of specific types of commodities, affect these indicators. We might then put to the test J. M. Clark's thesis that

> many a commodity commands a price merely because its negative social value [presumably, insofar as it is known] is less than the costs involved in suppressing its use ... [and that] ... exchange value will remain positive till the negative social value accumulates such overwhelming momentum as to stamp out the trade entirely.[32]

Going beyond specific products and their mode of production (and consumption), we must look at entire industries and even broader institutional aspects of our economy. If we regard our social institutions as means toward the furtherance of society's wellbeing (as indeed we should), then we need to study as, once more, Clark had recommended, "the particular economic gains and costs to society for which such institutions are responsible.[33]

Just one example, reflecting some of our current concerns, might serve as illustration. The problem complex of transportation, especially in urban areas, poses many unanswered questions and unexplored implications. Among the considerations that have a bearing is, first of all and rather obviously, the prime objective: the expeditious, safe, convenient, and economical movement of people. The prevailing reliance on private transportation by means of owner-driven family cars, in contrast to public transportation, has the *prima facie* plausibility, from the vehicle owner's point of view, of expeditiousness and convenience, with comparative safety and economy being, at best, open questions. The ongoing explorations of the externalities of the massive use of private transportation, notably the external dyseconomies of air pollution through the waste products of the burnt automobile fuel, are bringing to light a substantial cost factor that has been virtually completely ignored in previous calculations of costs and benefits. It must enter a broadened benefit-cost calculus, at least insofar as the factors of safety and economy are concerned.

However, a perceptive social accounting of causes and effects cannot stop there. It will have to broach the question of the extent to which primary reliance on privately owned motor vehicles has affected the availability and quality of public means of transport; and how the ensuing state of affairs has, in its turn, affected, e.g., the accessibility of labor markets in and outside the inner city for those without private cars, particularly those living in heavily populated, low-income areas. If an adverse cause-and-effect relationship is established, then—carrying the train of thought to its logical conclusion, yet by no means *ad absurdum*—one may raise questions such as the following: To what extent did the inconvenience and the high cost of public transport between the Watts district of Los Angeles and the locations in which its inhabitants could seek and find work have a share in causing the human frustrations which led to the Watts riots?[34] A social cost accounting of this comprehensive kind might shed altogether new light on the true total cost of the institution of owner-driven private transportation, at least in metropolitan communities.

It is immediately evident that much of the information required is not readily available, nor has the gathering and evaluation of such information traditionally been considered to lie within the domain of the economist. But this is precisely a part of the challenge of social economics: to broaden the input of economic analysis so as to take account of information not heretofore utilized but the relevance of which is coming to be recognized and which, as a consequence, will increasingly be sought after by stepping up coordinated research efforts across disciplinary lines.

Social Economics as a Link Between Social Ecology and Social Policy

The task which the foregoing subsection leads up to implies a perception of interlocking social relationships that far exceeds the present state of our knowledge. Yet, such knowledge should not be beyond our reach, nor is it as far "out" as it may appear at first sight. The framework within which these interlocking relationships work themselves out spans the remaining two dimensions of social economics in Hagenbuch's conceptual scheme: the study of social causes and social consequences of economic behavior. The concept of social ecology encompasses both and adds a further component—the notion of a system in which both are links in a continuous process that conforms to certain laws or rules to keep it in some sort of balance or equilibrium.

The analogy to the concept of ecology in nature is obvious and is intended. The relevance of this natural science concept to economists—far beyond all earlier imagining—has been driven home only recently in an article written by Ayres and Kneese, two researchers connected with Resources for the Future, Inc.[35] Discussing the nature of external dyseconomies associated with the disposal of residuals from the production and consumption process, the two authors point out that the creation of waste products and, hence, the problem of waste disposal are regular concomitants of that process. They take issue with the conventional view according to which consumption of the commodities produced marks a terminal phase. Instead, they represent the process as a circular flow of materials without a clear starting or ending point. Since, according to the laws of nature, matter is not destroyed but merely transformed, they stress that the disposal of wastes left from production and consumption processes in a way that will not hinder or impair the renewal process is of the essence. Thus, a crucial role for a nation's—and the world's—economy is seen to fall to the natural environment, viz., its capacity to absorb and transform the waste products so as not to upset this self-renewing cycle. This crucial role of the environment grows in proportion (and the capacity to perform it successfully assumes ever more critical portents) as the growth of population and technology begins to strain the absorptive capacity of finite natural resources that heretofore were thought to be—or have been treated as if they were—available in unlimited quantities.

In light of this insight, the analogy of social ecology can no longer be regarded as farfetched. The same trends that affect our natural environment, i.e., growing population density and advancing technology, unleash or accentuate impacts of human activities upon the social environment by extending their radius and intensifying their thrust. The analogy of a circular flow, though less apparent, becomes plausible in that the growing physical proximity enhances reactions and feedbacks. The corrosive quality of such accentuated conflicts of interest and the ensuing clashes—ever more openly displayed—is undeniable; and the growing incapacity of the social fabric to absorb the strain is reflected in their rising nonresolution, which enhances the rigidity of the opposing positions and depth of feeling, i.e., it feeds on itself. Remembering Galbraith's theory of social balance, it would appear that a far broader interpretation of this theory is not only permissible but called for, as the tolerance of the social system could be strained beyond the point of self-renewal.

It goes without saying that the arena in which the events and forces under reference unfold is far broader than that of economists. Many, probably most, of the insights needed will have to be obtained by social scientists in other disciplines, notably social psychologists, and by practitioners of various other skills, such as social workers and public health specialists. The duty and function of the economist—even the social economist, who is sensitized to the happenings in cognate fields—are limited. His legitimate and crucial role must be that of an analyst, diagnostician, and prognostician with regard to those phases of the continuous process where causes or results, i.e., actions or reactions, originate from or reverberate on the economic level or where there appears to be a reasonable expectation that they are susceptible to influence by economic moves.

In this connection, a crucial gap in our economic studies is worthy of note. It concerns the problem syndrome that covers, in a variety of forms, what might be termed disinvestment in man or, simply, the neglect of human resources. The common disregard of the economic consequences of this far-flung phenomenon is all the more surprising in view of the considerable recognition and attention the concept of investment in man and the measurement of its returns have received in recent years among economists.[36] Awareness of this long-ignored aspect of economic development and a proper appreciation of its important role in economic growth came about as a result of the discovery by Simon Kuznets, E. F. Denison, and others that our long-term economic growth was far greater than could be explained by the mere increase in capital and in man-hours worked. Thus, our attention was turned to the importance of upgrading human capabilities, and we came to view them as produced means of production, i.e., as a form of capital.[37] Not only education and training but also physical and mental health and many other aspects of human development that had long been viewed merely as consumption thus assumed a special role, more recently referred to as productive consumption or, simply, as investment.

But while, in recognition of this human-capital factor, we are prepared nowadays to credit better than half of our economic growth to such improvements (including know-how and technological advance), we have yet to turn our attention to past and presumable future losses due to our failure to develop the human potential and our either wanton or negligent destruction of human assets. In the 1950's, economists developed (and have since applied) the concept of full-employment output, i.e., the potential national product which the economy is capable of producing if all those seeking work are actually employed. Concomitantly, there was developed the concept of a full-employment budget, surplus or deficit, i.e., a public expenditure and taxation program designed so as to produce a balanced budget, a budget surplus, or a budget deficit, depending on which of these three possibilities was called for (along with other economic measures) to assure full employment while avoiding inflation. Although we have not as yet learned how to avoid either of these two evils without begetting the other, our commitment to a public economic policy that seeks to avoid both insofar as possible is beyond doubt.

What needs to be developed in the 1970's is a somewhat analogous, but more inclusive, concept of a full-performance budget, i.e., a performance goal premised on the release of the full human potential of our population. Such a target would not necessarily presuppose gainful employment as the ultimate objective for everyone not now in the labor market or even for all those now part of it. Rather, it would give expression to a planful, coherent, and sustained social policy of coming to grips with the several dysfunctional aspects of our society that sap its strength, narrow its economic base, and impose upon it substantial yet avoidable social costs.[38]

The role of the social economist as an adviser on public policy—especially in social policy matters—readily emerges as one of great potential significance. His ability to rise to the challenge that awaits him will require of him more than the mastery of the conventional skills and techniques of economics. Among the necessary extensions of his horizon is a new perception of the social ecology of disinvestment in man. It will have to occupy a central place. It must begin with the adverse consequences of malnutrition and other impairments of the health of expectant mothers, the lack of infant care, and child neglect, and range all the way to the stifling and stultifying results of the various all-too-common deprivations due to the denial of normal human needs of a suitable family (or suitable substitute) environment, a positive socialization (acculturation) and learning experience in preschool and school settings, an achievement orientation acceptable to society, and the acquisition of useful skills, opportunities for human growth and economic advancement—in short, all the major obstacles to individual self-realization and social acceptance will have to be taken into account. Available knowledge not now utilized and further knowledge about causes and effects yet to be produced by ecologists, medical and psychiatric researchers, psychologists, sociologists, criminologists, social workers and others will have to be tapped. Any known or newly discovered interconnections between, say, nutrition and learning ability, maternal care and infant health, child neglect or abuse and delinquency, overcrowding and aggression, will have to be translated into economic terms, i.e., "costed," by methods yet to be developed, and then applied in a much widened cost-benefit accounting by economists.

Viewed in this perspective, an important consideration in evaluating alternative public policies and programs (both preventive and remedial) will have to focus on the "opportunity social cost" (of not instituting such programs) rather than merely on the monetary savings due to less "costly" programs or no programs at all. The purview of social economics must extend beyond that traditional to welfare economics, because welfare economics, despite its long quest for a solid theoretical foundation of the maximization of welfare and, concomitantly, the optimum allocation of scarce economic resources, continues to be committed to the concept of a social welfare function that is derived through some elusive aggregation of individual preferences, even though some of its leading theoreticians have acknowledged that social determinants enter into individual value judgments.[39] Clark predicted the need for cross-disciplinary expansion of the horizon of economists beyond such self-contained social escapism:

> Economists can certainly not follow a policy of Jeffersonian nonintercourse toward other fields of knowledge. The ultimate problems in which humanity is interested are not those of social value in the sense of "value in society" as registered by market standards. Men are interested in values of things *to* society, and they rightly demand that economics should contribute to the solution of these problems.[40]

Having "inherited an economics of irresponsibility," Clark foresaw a "swing of the pendulum . . . toward a sense of solidarity and social-mindedness."[41] In the presence of social risks of overwhelming proportions, when we can no longer just assume that most men "could 'fall on their feet' whatever happened" but where "the consequences are too serious to be treated thus cavalierly . . . the environment has become responsible for John Smith. But at the same time John Smith has become responsible for the environment." To clinch his argument, he concluded that "many things are not be be taken for granted as of old because they are things over which someone can exercise control, and that means they are things for which someone is responsible."[42]

A new "economics of responsibility" may, indeed, be dawning. Its prime characteristic would be an admixture of genuine social concern along lines which were so aptly formulated, not long ago, by the Economic Council of Canada:

> The long-term record of the growth of material wealth in today's high income countries has been impressive. But this growth does not proceed without social costs, and it has been tending to throw into sharper focus a growing array of problems and needs relating to both the quality of life and to an appropriate sharing in the fruits of economic progress. Illustrative of the issues which have become the subject of increasing social concern are: the problem of poverty in the midst of affluence; the needs for better access to high standards of health care and to opportunities for maximum educational advancement for all individuals in the society; increased air and water pollution in an age of greatly advanced scientific capabilities for dealing with these problems; increased urban congestion and blight concentrated especially in centres of the highest average of income and wealth; and the greatly increased needs for recreational facilities and enlarged cultural opportunities in conditions of reduced working time and increased leisure. In these and other fields, there has emerged an increasing awareness that under conditions of high income and well sustained economic growth there are both needs and opportunities for devoting proportionately greater resources to the maintenance and improvement of the quality of life. More generally, there has also emerged a strong conviction that economic growth and development cannot be regarded as satisfactory if the rising output and income which it generates is not widely shared

among all groups and all parts of the country. A more equitable distribution of rising opportunities, income and wealth has thus become a more prominent objective of modern industrial economies along with other basic economic and social goals.[43]

Reading this, one may be reminded of an admonition from an altogether different source and time—John Donne's

> No man is an island, entire to itself; every man is a piece of the continent, a part of the main; ... any man's death diminishes me, because I am involved in mankind, and therefore never send to know for whom the bell tolls; it tolls for thee.

As happens so often, the poet or religious seer appears to have divined well in advance that which it takes the more earthbound explorer of the social scene a longer time to discover and unravel.

Notes

1. John Maurice Clark, "The Changing Basis of Economic Responsibility," written in 1916 and reprinted in his *Preface to Social Economics, Essays on Economic Theory and Social Problems* (New York, Farrar and Rinehart, 1936), p. 80.

2. This is not to say that the Classical economists were opposed to any and all kinds of government intervention in the national economy. For a comprehensive review of the types of government action that various exponents of the Classical school of economic liberalism deemed justified in certain fields and under certain conditions, see Lionel Robbins' essay, "The Economic Functions of the State," *The Theory of Economic Policy in English Classical Political Economy* (London: Macmillan, 1952), pp. 34-61; also reprinted in *Private Wants and Public Needs,* edited by E. S. Phelps (New York: W. W. Norton & Co., Revised edition, 1965), pp. 96-103. A more recent restatement of the Classical Liberal position, by Milton Friedman, in *Capitalism and Freedom* (Chicago: University of Chicago Press, 1962) would appear to draw the lines of acceptable government intervention much more narrowly; see especially the Preface and Chapters 1 and 2.

3. Clark, op. cit., p. 44.

4. Alvin H. Hansen, *The American Economy* (New York: McGraw-Hill, 1957), p. 146.

5. John Kenneth Galbraith, *The Affluent Society* (Boston: Houghton Mifflin, 1958).

6. Galbraith, op. cit., Chapters 9-11.

7. Ibid, Chapter 18. A convenient selection containing the passages here referred to can be found under the title "The Dependence Effect and Social Balance" in *Private Wants and Public Needs,* pp. 13-36.

8. Professor Galbraith himself came to acknowledge and emphasize this point in his later book *The New Industrial State* (Boston: Houghton Mifflin, 1967).

9. *Technology and the American Economy.* Report of the National Commission on Technology, Automation, and Economic Progress. Volume I, February 1966 (Washington, D.C.: U.S. Government Printing Office).

10. Op. cit., p. 96.

11. Ibid.

12. Ibid, pp. 96-97.

13. Quoted in the transmittal letter accompanying the product of this inquiry (see

below). *Toward A Social Report.* U.S. Department of Health, Education and Welfare. Washington, D.C., U.S. Government Printing Office, 1969, p. iii.

14. *Toward a Social Report, passim,* but especially the Introduction and the Appendix.

15. Ibid., p. 97.

16. Ibid, pp. 100-101.

17. Galbraith, "The Dependence Effect and Social Balance," p. 15.

18. See Ian McHarg, *Design with Nature* (Berryville, Va.: Doubleday & Co., 1969).

19. In the United States the term was used in the 1930's and occasionally thereafter; see, in addition to Clark, op. cit., Alvin S. Johnson, *Essays in Social Economics* (New York: New School for Social Research, 1954). More recently, it has been revived in a Brookings Institution series, titled "Studies in Social Economics." The works published in this series to date deal with problems of medical economics, education and poverty, and social security.

20. Walter Hagenbuch, *Social Economics,* Cambridge Economic Series, Cambridge, England, the University Press, 1958.

21. Alfred Marshall, *Principles of Economics,* 8th ed., 1920, p. 780, as quoted in Hagenbuch, *Social Economics,* op. cit., p. 1.

22. Hagenbuch, op. cit., p. 2.

23. Ibid.

24. Robert J. Lampman, "Toward an Economics of Health, Education and Welfare," *Journal of Human Resources,* vol. 1, no. 1 (Summer 1966), pp. 45-53. For an elaboration of some aspects of this categorization, see Dr. Lampman's opening essay in Part 2 of this book.

25. J. M. Clark, *Studies in the Economics of Overhead Costs,* (Chicago: University of Chicago Press, 1923), p. 16.

26. *Preface to Social Economics, op cit.,* p. 54.

27. Ibid., p. 45.

28. Hagenbuch makes reference to "social accounting" in discussing concepts of national income and product. (Cf. his *Social Economics,* pp. 15-19.)

29. Cf. *Indicators of Social Change,* edited by E. B. Sheldon and W. E. Moore, New York, Russel Sage Foundation, 1968, and *Social Indicators,* edited by Raymond A. Bauer, Cambridge, Mass., The M.I.T. Press, 1966.

30. *Indicators of Social Change, op. cit.,* p. 91.

31. Ibid., pp. 91 and 93.

32. Clark, *Preface to Social Economics,* p. 55.

33. Ibid., p. 65.

34. This question was actually raised, in essentially this form, by Michael Harrington at a Colloquium, "The Translation of Ideas and Knowledge into Action for the Welfare of Society," sponsored by the School of Applied Social Sciences of Case Western Reserve University in Cleveland, Ohio, in September, 1966. A somewhat generalized account is given in *Social Theory and Social Invention,* edited by Herman D. Stein (Cleveland: Press of Case Western Reserve University, 1968), pp. 52-53.

35. Robert U. Ayres and Allen V. Kneese, "Production, Consumption and Externalities," *American Economic Review, vol. 59, no. 3 (June 1969), pp. 282-297.*

36. See the pioneering work done by Theodore W. Schultz; also the writings of Gary S. Becker. For a brief exposition of several pertinent treatments, see "Investment in Human

Beings," *Journal of Political Economy,* vol. 70, no. 5 (October 1962), Part 2, Supplement. For a more recent collection of essays, see e.g., E. B. Jakubauskas and C. P. Baumol, eds., *Human Resources Development* (Ames: Iowa State University Press, 1967).

37. Schultz, op cit., p. 1.

38. Something of a beginning might be seen in the "Freedom Budget" developed by the A. Philip Randolph Institute (New York, October 1966, revised).

39. Cf. Kenneth J. Arrow: "The principle of extended sympathy as a basis for interpersonal comparisons seems basic to many of the welfare judgments made in ordinary practice. It remains to be seen whether an adequate theory of social choice can be derived from this and other acceptable principles" ("Public and Private Values" in *Human Values and Economic Policy,* edited by Sidney Hook, New York, New York University Press, 1967, p. 20); also James S. Doesenberry: "The view that preferences are a matter of individual personality alone is certainly untenable" (*Income, Saving and the Theory of Consumer Behavior,* Harvard Economic Studies, vol. 87, 1948, p. 112).

40. Clark, *Preface to Social Economics,* p. 61.

41. Ibid., p. 67.

42. Ibid., pp. 69-71.

43. Economic Council of Canada, *Third Annual Review: Prices, Productivity, and Employment* (Ottawa: Queen's Printer, November 1966), p. 21.

Part 2   Maximizing National Product While Meeting Social Needs

2

Economic Policy Objectives and Problem Areas

Robert J. Lampman

We in the United States today are concerned about many problem areas in our economy. We are concerned about the general rate of economic growth, about unemployment, about inflation and the balance of payments. We are concerned about poverty. We are concerned about the status of our black citizens. We are concerned about the quality and accessibility of health services. We are concerned about education and housing. We are concerned about family instability and the delinquency of some of our young people. We are concerned about air pollution and water pollution and about transportation. We are concerned about making modern living possible—to say nothing of making it enjoyable. And we are also concerned about ways to get people to participate in the matters that affect their destiny.

A Common Framework for the Economics of Health, Education and Welfare

All of those concerns might be thought of as economic problems or as having economic aspects. How to put them all into some general order and give a base for thinking about them is a great challenge. The Institute for Social Economics, which is being inaugurated at Temple University exemplifies one approach. I have thought for some time that we ought to have a subdiscipline of economics called economics of health, education and welfare, because it does seem there is a unity among the questions that are taken up in the study of health and the supply of medical care; of education and the supply of schooling, training and retraining, and hence, many of our manpower policies; of the redistribution of income by cash transfers through social insurance and public assistance.[1] They have a certain unity because the reallocations to health and education are intended to have redistributive effects, and the cash payments have reallocative effects. This means that in this area of social economics or whatever we want to call it, it is hard to separate allocative efficiency from distributional equity.

It is also true that in all three of these areas there is an unusual mix of private and public suppliers; there is a complex structure of demand associated with unusually uncertain outcomes; probabilistic events lie at the root of all calculations; and there are in each of these areas extraordinarily significant external benefits.

The economics of health, education, and welfare may be divided into two parts. One might say there are some things that are general in character and that affect all of us in a community setting—such things as transportation, broad community planning, and control of air and water pollution. There are others that are quite personal—the transfers to individuals of educational services, health services, and welfare payments, etc.

I don't know whether those determining policy for the new institute will define "social economics" in a similar way, but I do hope they will help to develop a framework within which our students can take hold of the interlocking set of questions that we all sense is involved.

Economic Goals

Let me now review briefly our economic goals and suggest that there are several ways of thinking about these goals. It is conventional to say that America's leading economic goals are, in the language of the Employment Act of 1946, maximum employment, production, and purchasing power. Moreover, it is widely understood that we have attained these goals to a degree unpredicted on the basis of our experience in the 1930's. Unemployment is about 3½ per cent of the labor force. Per capita product, which is about $4,500 a person, has increased about one half in real terms in twenty years. The purchasing power of the representative family, as measured by its price-adjusted consumption, has moved along in step with increased production.

So if one were Rip Van Winkle and had been asleep for twenty years, one might say that we have achieved most of our goals, that everything is going fine. But as you know, there is a malaise which attends all these achievements. Most immediately, this arises from the frustrations, uncertainties, and discords that surround our policy in Vietnam. Even though this has been a relatively small economic effort, taking only about 3 per cent of the gross national product—less than a year's growth in the economy—it is an effort that has raised the deepest issues of national purpose.

There is also a lot of anxiety among people about the persistent deficit in our balance of payments. This deficit has recently moderated, but the possibility of speculation against the dollar and a breakdown of international exchange is a very real worry to many people. Many critics on the right believe that our prosperity is not soundly based and cannot long prevail. They allege that not only have we been living beyond our international means but that recent increases in domestic private and public debt and commitments of future income to expanding social welfare programs cannot be sustained. Associated with this gloomy outlook is the belief that our post-World War II economic success has been forced by the artificial demands of a cold-hot war mix and could not otherwise have been managed.

I am often asked by people, "When are we going to have good times again?" They don't really believe that what we have now is prosperity. I think this stems very often from their concern about debt and about the increasingly great role of the government in the economy.

Certainly, many careful observers believe that our prosperity, while it may be real, has brought us many problems that we don't know how to solve or are unwilling to solve. The rapid migration from farms and from small towns to metropolitan areas has brought racial turmoil and crises in transportation, education, and environmental control. And some critics say that while these public problems fester, we give higher priority to less important needs of affluent private consumers.

At the same time, looking now to the left, the host of postwar babies now coming of age challenge us to live up to our professed goals—and often these are goals that had higher priorities in the days before the Great Depression—and give them new opportunities. I am sure many of you have been struck by the fact that the goals of many New Leftists sound like old-fashioned conservatism. They believe in a much diminished role for government. They are not easily persuaded that this is the best of all possible worlds or that the Employment Act encompasses the most important purposes for society. Indeed, they often respond affirmatively to the allegation that the economic system, which they see as dominated by an oligarchic establishment, is a central part of a sick society that produces distorted personalities and broken communities.

Kenneth Boulding recently said that one of the biggest problems for our economy is people's rising expectations. Many youngsters today are Utopian in their views. They consider what we have achieved to date as somehow barbaric and they talk about much better things ahead. Mr. Boulding suggested that what we need most of all is a revolution of falling expectations. Everything would be better if we just didn't expect so much.

In quick summary, then, at this point we can say that America's achievement of what are often called its leading economic goals is now challenged by critics ranging from the old right to the new left, all of whom assert that we have been pursuing the wrong goals or assigning the wrong priorities to them.

Types of Goals

Now I would like to ask you to take a closer look at the types of goals we have. One way to identify goals is in terms of questions that are familiar to all of you who have taught elementary economics. These are, what is going to be produced? how is it going to be produced? who is going to get the product? what is the level of activity and output to be?

In broad terms, we answer these questions as follows: "What?" is answered by an allocation of 65 per cent of the total product to meet the demands of private consumers; 20 per cent to government, with one-half of that for national defense; and 15 per cent to business for replacing and expanding the stock of capital goods and inventories and houses.

The question of how the product is produced is answered primarily by the term "privately," with less than 10 per cent of the product originating in the government sector.

Who gets the product is determined in largest part by the answers to the two previous questions. In other words, income is distributed in response to production, which responds in turn to market demands. About three fourths of income is in the form of wages and salaries; one fourth is property income in the form of profits, rent, and interest. These producer incomes are, of course, shared with family members who are not productive. Moreover, about 7 per cent of income is collected in taxes for transfer in the form of social insurance, public assistance, and related cash benefits. In addition to these cash benefits, a set of service benefits—the most important being education—are distributed by public institutions without regard to current productivity of the beneficiaries.

This system of transfer of money and services has been growing faster than total product, of which it now comprises about one sixth.[2] In 1967 it amounted to $132 billion worth of transfers. Not all of this transferring is from rich to poor; some of it is from the poor to the rich, and some from the middle class to the middle class. But using the term "transfer" very broadly, we are talking about a very big part of our total product. One sixth is more than we spend on national defense. It is more than we spend on a lot of other things. I think that this suggests at least part of the scope of study for an institute of social economics.

Arising out of all of this is a distribution of income that is moderately unequal compared with that of other countries. The degree of inequality is somewhat less than obtained before World War II, but it does not appear to have declined since the end of the war. With income inequality unchanged and average income rising, it is not surprising that the proportion of the population in poverty has been falling. In 1969 only about 23 million people, or 11 per cent of the total population, were in poverty, as defined by the Social Security Administration's classification of poverty-line incomes. That figure has been dropping recently at the rate of more than 2 million per year. Maintaining that rate of poverty reduction is a feasible goal for our economy.

Level of Activity

The level of activity is another leading question for our economy. This, of course, is influenced by a wide range of private and public decision-makers. The overall growth rate for the potential to produce has recently shifted from about 3 per cent to 4 per cent a year. The shift is due mostly to an acceleration of growth in the labor force, but it is due partly to an improvement of efficiency in converting raw inputs to final outputs. With increases of labor running at 1.7 per cent per year, increases of capital at 3 per cent, and increases of land at 0 per cent, it is estimated that over half of the increased output remains to be explained by improvements in the quality of labor—human resources, if you want to call it that—and capital, technology, economies of scale, and organization and management.[3] Here, again, we are touching on the field of social economics.

The federal government's fiscal and monetary policies are aimed at keeping overall demand in line with the increasing potential to produce. There is widespread agreement that government should compensate for the discrepancies between potential output and demand for such output which appear from time to time. This, of course, is "the new economics," which has given us one of the great social breakthroughs of the 20th century; and we now have some reason to be confident that with careful management we can avoid great depressions and runaway inflation. There is perhaps less agreement that taxes and credit policies should be designed to improve the rate of capital formation and, hence, the potential to produce.

Classification of Goals

Process Goals. Much of the discussion of economic goals has to do with processes. The pure types of economic process, as Robert Heilbroner lays them out, are the traditional, the market, and the centrally directed.[4] A traditional society is typified by the prenational economy of feudalistic Europe. A centrally directed society is exemplified by the Soviet Union. In a pure market society, which is approximated by the United States, individuals are released from traditional status bonds that hold them to one place, one employer, and one style of life. No central authority specifies what they must do to fulfill a national plan. Rather, they are left free to make contracts for their work, to buy and sell land and other property, and to direct the pattern of final output by their consumer decisions.

The American economy's processes are a mix of tradition direction, central direction, and market direction. Yet the greater part of our value load is supportive of market processes and the individualism associated with them. Thus the Employment Act specifies that the employment and production goals are to be pursued "in a manner calculated to foster and promote free competitive enterprise and the general welfare."

In our society the powers of government are limited, and success or failure in reaching economic objectives turns on the energies and initiative of our citizens in their capacities as businessmen, workers, and farmers. Government provides a basic framework within which such choices are to be made, sometimes limiting the range of the permissible, sometimes enlarging the range of the feasible. Maximizing the free choices effectively open to all individuals is the basic aim of economic policy in a democracy, where ultimate value is the integrity and dignity of the individual human being. In the pure market rhetoric, the goal of developing worthwhile human beings is realizable only where individuals are free to make their own decisions and to bear the responsibility for those decisions. The prime values are freedom and opportunity. Novelty and change are facilitated; familiar ways of doing things and security are downgraded. Rewards go to the quick and the responsive, rather than to the loyal and the old-fashioned.

The consistent spokesman for the market process defends it in terms of character-building rather than as a way to build GNP, and would stand by it even though it could be demonstrated that it did less for national production than central direction. The striving is more important than the achieving. John Stuart Mills' essays are illustrative of this view. In this system of thought, economic goals of the nation are the sum of the goals of individuals, and whatever production and consumption patterns arise are by definition the right patterns. They are validated by consumer sovereignty, on the one hand, and competitive discipline, on the other hand.

It is a commonplace to observe that we have departed from, if indeed we were ever fully committed to, the pure market process. The liberal system gave people not only the freedom to compete but also the freedom to combine. Americans have sought, by means of the large-scale business corporation, tariffs, labor unions, trade and professional associations, and social legislation, to moderate the rigors of the market. They have sought group security and limits on inequality of opportunity and condition. But in these departures from the pure market process, they have not gone far toward central direction. Decisions are still made in a decentralized, pluralistic, check-and-balances fashion, and no single person or group can act definitively on many issues.

Our process goals have tended to favor individual and voluntary group decisions. However, this preference has not denied a role for government in regulating relationships between buyer and seller, employer and employee, and landlord and tenant, nor in promoting business and providing key services for economic and social development. These roles for government are legitimized by the democratic process and are seen as ways to harmonize conflicting goals of producer and consumer groups. Ideally, they leave considerable room for minorities and do not overrule the most deeply held values of any group. The aim of the several parties is to bargain with but not liquidate the partners in the enterprise. We have, in other words, what Selig Perlman calls a collective-bargaining state rather than a class-oriented state.[5]

One other way of thinking about process goals is suggested by looking at the matter of transfers. Many people are as concerned with the process used in developing a cash-transfer system as they are with the actual results. The different processes may be considered as three mentalities. One is what I would call an income tax mentality; a second is the minimum-provision mentality; and the third, the social-fault mentality.

The income tax mentality looks at the whole set of transfers from the point of view of horizontal and vertical equity, trying to bring some order into our patchwork system of taxing, on the one hand, and paying out cash benefits, on the other. I have noticed that a person who is carefully trained in income taxation is horrified when he begins to examine our system for paying out money. He can't find either vertical or horizontal equity, and this troubles him a great deal. So the natural thing for him to recommend in looking at the future is NIT, as a way of bringing symmetry into the overall system.

The minimum-provision mentality comes to us out of the concept of public assistance. It is based on the idea that some who have unmet needs have a certain claim upon the community. This is the emphasis behind in-kind transfer programs and child allowances, for example.

The social-fault mentality places responsibility for damages on the party best able to prevent the accident and best able to pay. Social fault theories gained expression, of course, in workmen's compensation, where the focus was on accidents, and they also underly unemployment compensation and old age and survivor benefits. The concentration on insurance against loss means that benefits are apt to be less than needed for low income families and that, in fact, benefits may be redistributed from the poor to the rich.

It is interesting to note that experts who start with different emphases are apt to raise quite different issues of horizontal equity, vertical redistribution, and benefit adequacy. So I would cite this as an example of how we often spend a lot of time talking about processes when we are thinking about economic policy and goals.

Overall-Performance Goals. Quite distinct from the process goals are what we may define as the overall-performance goals we have for our economy. These have been emphasized more in recent times than they were earlier in history. These goals are national, rather than individual, in character and involve total employment, aggregate production, general price levels and the balance of payments. As President Kennedy put it in his famous "economic myths" speech at Yale University in 1962, "The national interest lies in high employment and steady expansion of output, in stable prices and a strong dollar."[6] In that speech he urged that we not be doctrinaire about preferred processes in seeking ways to achieve important performance goals. These goals, he said, cannot be reached by "incantations from the forgotten past." He might also have said that they cannot be reached by decentralized processes alone and that they require a strong head at the center.

It can be argued, of course, that these performance goals are supportive, rather than destructive, of our process goals, which are basically justified in terms of their contribution to the ultimate goals of freedom and their challenge to individuals. Achievement of the performance goals enlarges the range of choice and opportunity for individuals. Some of the same justification may hold for the goals of social security and of the war on poverty, and so on; that is, we are trying to enlarge the opportunity for people to do what they choose.

Specific-Use-of-Output Goals. Overall performance goals are more concrete than process goals, and what we can call specific-use-of-output goals are more concrete than either. Here we are talking about specific accomplishments, such as better housing, trips to the moon, new urban transit systems, regional medical centers, and preschool and postschool training. We are talking, as the National Planning Association (NPA) would have us do, of a national economic budget that shows all expenditures, private and public, classified by object and purpose of expenditure.

Going beyond process goals and performance goals to more specific goals is justified, some believe, by the assertion that there is a national, as well as an individual and local, interest in the achievement of high standards in education, health, and research and development. It is not surprising that the NPA estimates that our aspirations for the year 1975 in 16 such fields, which were defined to be all-inclusive, would have a cost well in excess of the total GNP expected for that year.[7] Hence, even though our current prosperity continues, priorities will need to be set. We have had a lot of change in our goals, and especially in our thinking about performance goals and specific uses of output. Over the years our goals have gained in specificity and in the degree to which they are national in character.

Selecting and Achieving Goals

How should we think about goals? What can we, as scholars, do to help citizens and policy-makers intelligently select and reach goals?

Descriptive Analysis

Clearly, the first thing that we all need is a descriptive analysis of the American economy that gives attention to the problems to which policies are addressed. For example: How many people are unemployed? How long have they been umemployed? Who and where are they? It may call attention to new problems as they arise. As Bertrand de Juvenel says, "Designers of statistics are indeed philosophers, however unwilling to claim the name, and are fully aware that different aspects of reality can be lit up if alternative sets of concepts are used."[8] On the other hand, as Bertram Gross points out:

> It is often the case that our intelligence machinery tends to creak along in bureaucratic conformance with routine set up in a previous era. Our conservative defenders of the status quo rarely see much of the state at which we are. Our radical attackers of the present system (or power structure or establishment) are usually blind to the radical changes already taking place.[9]

One way that we can do descriptive analysis is illustrated by my notion about the American system of transfers. Let me suggest a new sort of social accounting for a $132 billion total of transfers for the United States in 1967.[10] Suppose we think about transferring as taking place in eight stages.

One stage is the increase of factor incomes by subsidizing earners. A wage subsidy or a farm subsidy may change factor income and hence change the distribution of income.

Second is the privately insured benefits financed by employers. This is a way of altering the distribution of income from what it would be if those benefits were paid in cash wages.

Third is tax-financed public cash and in-kind transfers. Here are the general set of social security, public assistance, education, and other in-kind programs. That adds up to $100 billion all by itself.

Fourth is employee-financed group and individual private insurance benefits. That's about $10 billion.

Fifth is certain reductions in market price, due to subsidy. These are consumer subsidies, such as rent supplements and food subsidies.

Sixth is transfers by a philanthropic institution—private institutions— churches, for example, and foundations.

Finally, we have gifts from one family to another, and gifts within the household to secondary units.

These all add up to $132 billion worth of transferring; and this is an example, I would say, of the kind of descriptive analysis or work which is sometimes helpful in thinking about our social policy.

Predictive Analysis

Beyond descriptive work, we need predictive analysis concerning how the system will or will not respond to the problems that are detected in description. This often calls for more than projection of past trends. It often necessitates theorizing about the motives and capabilities of such economic actors as workers, consumers, business firms, bankers. From such analysis one can hope to gain an understanding of which problems will yield to our standard processes or to nurture of overall performance goals, and which will need more specialized attention.

One example of predictive analysis work that we are engaged in at Wisconsin, in cooperation with a group at Princeton, is an experiment with negative income taxation. We are concerned with a thousand families in New Jersey who are to be subject to different treatments, so-called. They are being used as guinea pigs in trying to understand how people respond to different types of cash payments and different types of marginal tax rates that affect their income.

Array of Methods

A third thing we need to do is to conceive of an array of methods that may be useful in mitigating or solving a particular problem. And here I am pointing to cost-benefit analysis and program-planning budgeting as the wave of the future. The cost of the several methods for solution should be compared, accounting not only for resources to be used but for sacrifices to be made in terms of other goals. This means that, to some extent, a benefit-cost ratio for a particular method will depend upon the values of the social analyst. Hence, the policy-maker must himself use these ratios with an understanding of what, in fact, lies behind them.[11]

Cost Effectiveness

In principle, at least, the lines for rational decision-making are clear. The preferred methods for solving each of several problems are selected on the basis of cost effectiveness. Problems are ranked in terms of priority. The outlays are then allocated in such a way that the last dollar of outlay on each problem produces the same addition to social utility. This assumes that there are never enough resources completely to solve all problems, foreign and domestic, and that the issue then is to select the highest priority uses.

I believe that our capacity to solve problems is increasing over time, so it is part of the dynamics of the system that we have before us an agenda of unattained goals which invites attention from numerous private, as well as public, agencies and that we will come to these in some orderly way. Sometimes just the careful statement of a problem and the calculation of a very low benefit-to-cost ratio for all known methods is enough to call forth from unexpected quarters approaches that will prove feasible. We do have potentialities for social invention in this country, as well as for other types of invention.

Perhaps merely stating that all this descriptive work, predictive work and benefit-to-cost ratio work are needed is enough to indicate the impossibility of their achievement, even though we have the Institute for Social Economics and other institutes like it around the country. No one person or organization can comprehend so much about so many processes and relationships. The best that we can do is to make some progress toward some of our goals a bit at a time. To do so will require continuing and thoughtful effort at the several levels of private and public decision-making. It will require that different groups assume responsibility for various parts of what is needed.

I do have faith that we can meet these requirements to some degree and that our pragmatic American system will continue to fulfill substantial parts of an evolving set of economic goals.

Notes

1. Robert J. Lampman, "Toward an Economics of Health, Education and Welfare," The Journal of Human Resources, vol. 1, no. 1, 1966.

2. This "system" is discussed in Lampman, "Transfer and Redistribution as Social Process," in Alfred E. Kahn, editor, *Social Security in International Perspective* (Columbia University Press, forthcoming).

3. Edward F. Denison, *The Sources of Economic Growth in the United States and the Alternatives Before Us* (New York: Committee for Economic Development, 1962).

4. Robert L. Heilbroner, *The Making of Economic Society*. New York: Prentice-Hall, 1962.

5. "A Collective Bargaining Theory of the State," *Annals of the American Academy of Political and Social Science,* September 1946.

6. June 11, 1962. For an interesting discussion of the ideas set forth in this speech, see James Tobin, "The New Era of Good Feeling Between Business and Government," Chapter 4 in his *National Economic Policy* (New Haven, Conn.: Yale University Press, 1966).

7. Leonard A. Lecht, *Goals, Priorities, and Dollars* (New York: Free Press, 1966).

8. Cited by Bertram M. Gross and Michael Springer in "New Goals for Social Information," *Annals of the American Academy of Political and Social Science,* September 1967.

9. Ibid. Relevant here is the discussion surrounding Senator Walter F. Mondale's proposed Full Opportunity and Social Accounting Act, which would set up a council of social advisers to parallel the Council of Economic Advisers.

10. Lampman, "Transfer and Redistribution as Social Process."

11. See Robert Dorfman, editor, *Measuring Benefits of Government Investments* (Washington, D.C.: Brookings, 1965); and Samuel B. Chase, Jr., *Problems in Public Expenditure Analysis* (Washington, D.C.: Brookings, 1968).

3

Improving the Nation's Health: Joint Leverage for Economic and Social Adjustment

Gerard Piel

Were I to fulfill the assignment set for me and devote this discussion to "Improving the Nation's Health," then my survey would have to embrace the entire agenda projected for the three symposia in social economics scheduled for 1969.

Under the rubric of social economics, we should not be concerned merely to calculate the advantages of health in relation to increases in the gross national product. On the contrary, we should attempt to develop a more disciplined and structured notion of what it means to pursue the improvement of the nation's health as a social end in itself. We take for our objective nothing less than that framed for the World Health Organization (WHO): the realization and enjoyment by every human being of his and her full physiological and psychological potential.

Health, Medicine, and Social Progress

It is important to note that there is thus a distinction between health and medicine. When we define health as the founders of WHO did, medicine comes near the last of all the measures we would consider in the pursuit of health as a social value. Let me illustrate that statement by a brief review of the experience of our society with medicine since the turn of the century.

The life expectancy of the American population has increased in this time from forty-seven to seventy years. The crude death rate has been all but cut in half, from 17.2 per thousand population in 1900 to 9.6 per thousand in 1960 (see Figure 1). The age-adjusted death rate shows an even greater decrease: from 18 to 7.6 per thousand (see Figure 2). These figures are

Figure 1

Crude Death Rates: United States 1900-60

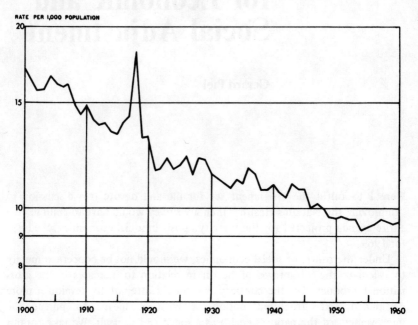

RATE PER 1,000 POPULATION

Source: *The Change in Mortality Trend in the United States,*
National Center for Health Statistics, Series 3 No. 1,
Washington, D. C., 1964

Figure 2

Age-Adjusted Death Rates: United States 1900-60

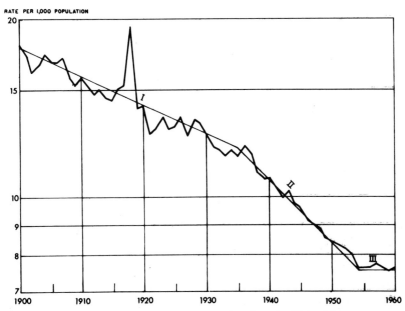

Source: *The Change in Mortality Trend in the United States,*
National Center for Health Statistics, Series 3 No. 1,
Washington, D. C., 1964

cited again and again in testimony to the miracle of modern medicine. When we plot the curve from 1900, however, we get an entirely different view of the social processes that brought this gain in human life.

The curve for the age-adjusted death rate shows three distinct slopes. The story of this succession affirms the distinction between medicine and health. Over the first thirty-five years the age-adjusted death rate declined from 18 to 12 per thousand; that is 80 per cent of the gain to 1960. Throughout the period from 1900 to 1935, medicine as we celebrate it today played a negligible role; there was little that the physician in face-to-face contact with his patient could do. It was, rather, the public health officer who made medicine's contribution to this development. The cleanup of water supplies, sewage disposal, food inspection, installation of indoor plumbing, and other developments in modern urban technology undoubtedly contributed even more heavily to the reduction of the death rate. These called for a still wider range of professional and engineering competence.

Ultimately, the decline in the death rate represents a summary expression of the nation's total economic growth and of the increase in the material well-being of the population.

This point is sharply illustrated by a statistical perception that we owe to Walsh McDermott. In 1900, 25 per cent of the deaths in the population were infant deaths. Of the infant deaths, half were caused by the so-called infant diarrheas and pneumonias. For these diseases, medicine has no specific remedies today. John Boyd-Orr, the founder of the Food and Agriculture Organization, identifies their real causes. "The one," he says, "is caused by bad feeding and the other by bad housing!"

In the poor countries of the world, these diseases continue to cause half of all infant deaths, which contribute heavily to the high death rates. In our country the two diseases have dwindled away. They declined with the birth rate, in the first place, and their decline coincides with the percolation of physical well-being down through the income groups to the very bottom. Today these diseases are isolated in the enclaves of the most wretched of our urban and rural slums. They still turn up, however, in the municipal hospitals of New York City and, I suppose, in Philadelphia and other cities.

In the second phase in the improvement of the nation's health, from 1935 to 1955, we see the effects of medicine, administered in the face-to-face physician-patient relationship. Between 1935 and 1955 the crude death rate declined from 12 to 7.6 per thousand. If this decline does not seem a large one, the new power of medicine still shows up plainly in the steeper slope of the age-adjusted curve. That curve descends at .15 per cent per annum up to 1935. It steepens then by a whole 60 per cent to an average decline of .22 per cent per annum from 1935 to 1955. During this period, of course, chemotherapy came to eliminate the infectious diseases from first rank among the causes of death in our population. There were other victories, like the polio vaccine. In the slope of the curve, however, the elimination of polio shows up scarcely at all. Yet to the parents of children who have grown up since 1954 this success, alone, looms larger than the 80 per cent decrease in the death rate accomplished before 1935.

In the third and present phase of the evolution of our vital statistics in this century, the death rate has flattened out. Since the mid-1950's it has run parallel to the base line, hovering within one or two tenths around the average of 7.6 per thousand. The oscillations reflect primarily the incidence of influenza from year to year. That ought to impress on our minds the caution that the vaunted conquest of the infectious diseases is not yet complete.

The reduction of infectious diseases has now brought organic afflictions to the fore. The American people live long enough to die of old age. The diseases of the heart and circulatory system and cancer account for more than half of all the deaths in our population. So, today, heart disease, cancer, and stroke are delimited as a new frontier of American life. Federal legislation has summoned the medical profession to curb, in the language of President Lyndon Johnson, "these killers." The cost of this massive program is yet to be reckoned, and the benefits will not be calculated for many years to come; whether the effort will have any effect whatever on the death rate cannot now be predicted.

Still, we can forgive people for wanting to live forever. Having made that concession to the impulse to immortality, however, we must consider whether a 9.6 per thousand crude death rate is not approaching the irreducible limit.

Closer study shows there is room for progress, for almost as much progress, perhaps, as was won from 1935 to 1955. The National Center for Health Statistics of the National Institutes of Health has examined the age-specific death rates in countries enjoying comparable benefits of industrial civilization. Choosing the best experience of each of the sixteen or so countries that are ahead of the United States by the standard of the crude death rate, the National Center put together a synthetic curve that brings the death rate down to as low as 7.3 per thousand.

When we compare the American experience with the most favorable experience from one age group to the other and from one cause of death to another in each of the other countries (and it was all carefully worked out in this study), we see some of the reasons why our country trails other countries in the attainment of the objectives for which we spend such a big portion of our national income. It comes as a shock, for example, to discover that just about the worst gap between the United States and other civilized countries—between our experience and the experience of all sixteen industrial countries in the study—appears in the infant death rate.

If we then consult the interior detail of our vital statistics we see the reason for this discrepancy. The infant death rates for the nonwhite population, wherever they are recorded in this country, run twice that of the white. That is true in New York City; the infant death rate doubles on the wrong side of 110th Street. Since color is so inextricably identified with poverty, we can deduce something (though our national statistics do not give us hard data for it) about the role that family income plays in the life and health experience of the disadvantaged members of our population. There is some direct evidence from other independent smaller studies. Paul Densen was able to demonstrate for the Health Insurance Plan of Greater New York not only the correlation of high infant death rate to low income but also to low quality of medical care.

In the higher mortality rates for all causes that prevail among the American poor, of whatever color, we can find a strategy for bringing the crude death rate of the U. S. population down from 9.6 to 7.3 per thousand. The figures show that if we could subtract the poverty-specific death rates from the U. S. experience we could, in round numbers, bring the death rate down close to the 7.3 per thousand figure confected from the best experience elsewhere in the world.

On the other hand, it is perfectly clear, we must bear in mind the distinction between health and medicine. By the application of the best medical care available we could not do much about the infant death rate of our poor. The infant death rate and the rate of premature delivery have a great deal more to do with the height-weight ratio of the adolescent unmarried mother who bears a child than with the kind of medical care she happens to have the luck to get. The intervention of medicine in the first trimester of her pregnancy is not going to do much about the blight already laid on the child in her womb.

But medicine is not totally irrelevant to our deliberations. We can usefully consider ways in which improvement in the health services can contribute to the nation's health.

New Institutions and Arrangements
in Medical Technology

In this exercise in social economics let me grasp the nettle instantly: The market process cannot effectively organize the technology of medicine for service to the individual or to the community.

The creation of the necessary new institutions and arrangements to make medical technology effective must begin with a complete reconstruction of the relations between private voluntary initiative, on the one hand, and public authority, on the other. Needless to say, as we proceed to consider the questions that are posed, events are already in motion and are moving outside of deliberate and rational control. The fat is already in the political fire, because the amendments of the 1965 Social Security Act—Medicare and Medicaid which stand with all credit to Wilbur Cohen and his colleagues—embody the worst features of the prevailing institutional and economic arrangements for the delivery of medical care in our country.

That legislation, to begin with, dumped hundreds of millions of new federal dollars into the fee-for-service private medical economy. The insurance feature of the legislation, reinforcing the established pattern of medical insurance in our country, places every conceivable obstacle in the way of preventive—which is to say accessible and early—medical care. The system, now so powerfully reinforced by federal dollars, promotes resort to the most costly modes of care: hospitalization and surgery. The welfare features in Medicaid exert the same economic bias in favor of acute episodic care. That welfare legislation also interposes the obnoxious means test between the patient and the care he needs, setting up psychological and moral hurdles to the accessibility of care.

Within a year of the passage of this legislation, the surfacing of unmet need and the inflation of prices in the medical marketplace brought such a huge excess of expense over prior estimates that the folk economists in Washington and in every state capital in the country turned around to cut back the benefits originally provided and to reduce the availability of what remained. The reverberation from that welching on a long-overdue public undertaking is now moving from the legislature into public consciousness.

Former Medicaid beneficiaries are once again being rejected by the voluntary hospitals that were so glad to welcome them when their human need came under escort by federal money. The big voluntary hospitals are sending these people back where they came from, that is, to the municipal hospitals.

We scarcely needed the present crisis to demonstrate the failure of the market process. Even in the bad old days—when medicine could not do its patients much good, when it was highly portable and available to the community in a black bag, and when it even made house-calls—the theoretically self-regulating economic mechanism did not secure the delivery of care to all people in the community. Charity filled the gaps. The modern hospital, as all must know, had its origin as a refuge for the poor. In our country, self-respecting middle-class people used to die at home. Early in the nineteenth century, in the cities of our eastern seaboard, it became socially unacceptable to have people dying on the sidewalk, as they do today in the great cities of the Southern Hemisphere. So the first hospitals were organized by charitable-religious people. The open ward was standard accommodation in these first hospitals. The private room did not figure in the design of hospitals until medicine and surgery had services to offer that required the workshops we know as the modern hospital.

This was the beginning of the caste system in medical care, with one kind of care for the paying customer and another for the charity patient. Under this system, conscientious physicians doubtless gave, and give today, their charity practice as much of their devotion as they give to their income-yielding patients. But caste distinction was and is nonetheless imposed by disparity in the physical circumstances in which care is rendered and by the moral circumstance that submits the charity patient to treatment as teaching and research "material." In connection with the launching of Medicare and Medicaid, it was instructive to hear the dismayed question from members of our medical faculties: "How are we ever going to train surgeons without the necessary teaching material?"

But ability to pay for medical care bears no natural connection with the care that people need. All the vital statistics insist that the relationship is, in fact, the reverse.

And in this relationship is the ethical disjunction; the U.S. medical economy becomes disjoined from the needs that it is bound, someday, to serve. For the present, the system of medical care prevailing in our country embodies, above all, the satisfaction of its beneficiaries on the two sides of the fee-for-service, free-choice-of-physician arrangement. This system is wonderfully designed to manage acute, episodic, and unusual diseases and injuries. Understandably, the crises of disease and injury take absolute precedence in the consumer's budget; for the worst crises the well-off are ready to spend the most. So correspondingly, the most richly rewarded in the highest-paying learned procession are those physicians and surgeons trained to cope with the severest and the rarest afflictions.

In order to prepare the medical student for the opportunity of rendering such service, our medical schools concentrate on a particular kind of medicine. As Willard Rappleye has observed, the afflictions that are the object of the principal outlay of treasure and talent in our medical schools constitute only a small segment of the total spectrum of the health problems of the population. The sensitive senior medical student also notes that the interesting cases on the ward are vastly outnumbered by the crocks. In preparation for the rough-and-tumble of competition in the market, however, he can tackle only a small segment of the total spectrum.

Without doubt, the system that functions under these extremes of social and economic pressure has produced care of extraordinary perfection and efficacy for those portions of the population that it serves and reaches. When we look at vital statistics, however, the evidence suggests that this system has not played as significant a role in the general improvement of the public's health as has the over-all steady growth of our economy as a whole.

In recent years, with the cost of medical care increasing along with its effectiveness, charity has yielded to welfare in the financing of the delivery of care to the medically indigent. Under the terms of the present arrangement between the government and the private economy, public authority is limited to filling the gaps, as charity did in the preceding decades. Public funds now go, therefore, to perpetuate the caste system in medical care.

The Medical Economy of New York City

In New York City we can see the caste system working at its optimum. The New York patriciate—that is to say, the grandsons and granddaughters of the next-to-last immigration wave—has always managed to maintain a close working understanding with the leadership of the last wave of immigration. In consequence, that city has historically devoted a larger percentage of its income to social services than any other big city in our country. Instead of the single giant county hospital that represents the public sector in most big American cities, the City of New York operates a chain of municipal hospitals which in 1969 numbered twenty-one and represented one-third of all the hospital beds in the city, plus a patchwork of clinics and neighborhood health service centers.

Norah Piore, the foremost student of the New York medical economy, has shown that the city treasury was footing one-third of the total bill for health services in New York City long before Medicaid was proffered to the nation. That one-third of the total outlay provided the health services received by 40 per cent of the population. It paid for half of all the patient-days in the hospitals, for the delivery of half of all the babies born in New York, for such pediatric services as were available to half of all the children in the city, and for the in-hospital and nursing-home care of perhaps 80 per cent of the elderly. Nor was there any stinting of expenditure. The city's outlay for its medical dependents exceeded by far the national average expenditure per capita.

The most recent appraisal of the working of this system was that produced by the Commission on Delivery of Personal Health Services that Mayor Lindsay got me to organize and conduct for him. Our findings can be summed up in the statement that the services provided are substandard, but that the services *not* provided—the gaps that remain unfilled—constitute the real failure of the personal health services of New York City. The New York experience, I am sure, constitutes a model of the rest of our land. For our big cities are all on their way to joining up in vast conurbations or megalopolises like New York.

In the New York City hospitals, first-rate professional services are available under the most wretched moral and physical conditions. The same service is available under better conditions in the larger voluntary hospitals that render much of the care that is paid for by the City. For lack of ambulatory care facilities and services, however, the medical problems presented at the municipal hospitals and on the wards of the voluntary hospitals are far more acute and difficult than those encountered in private and semi-private accommodations. That, of course, is why the poor make such good teaching material.

The out-patient departments and, over the last few years, the emergency rooms of the municipal hospitals are the principal site for the practice of pediatrics in New York. At eight o'clock at night in a New York City municipal hospital the benches in the emergency room are filled not by bloody heads from street fights and traffic accidents, but by mothers with their babies—mothers who have been waiting there since five o'clock and who could only get their kids there after they themselves got home from work.

For lack of adequate chronic care facilities, the wards upstairs in the municipal hospitals are filled with the elderly—people who do not belong in an acute general hospital and for whom the experience of life on a neglected ward is neither supportive nor therapeutic.

The psychiatric wards and services of all of the hospitals in the city still serve primarily as staging areas for shipping the emotionally ill to custodial care in state hospitals.

These failures cannot be charged to the City of New York, to its government, alone; they must be charged, as well, to the private medical economy. The allocation of resources to medical care in accord with the distribution of effective demand leaves gaps. In attempting to fill these gaps, the city is unable to outbid its competition for the resources it needs. Against the purchasing power and higher fiscal flexibility of the institutions in the voluntary sector, the city cannot hire doctors or nurses, to begin with. There is, therefore, not much that the city can do with what little else—the hospitals and other hardware—that it can buy, especially when it must buy that little too late.

The failure of the health services of the City of New York affects not only the welfare of the poor—not only the city's dependents on relief and not only the medically indigent bottom half of the population—but the welfare of the entire population as well. There was a good deal of misunderstanding and uninformed outrage around the country at the $6,000 annual-income standard that qualified a family of four for health services under the original Medicaid legislation passed by the State of New York. In point of fact, the health services of the city had long recognized a somewhat higher threshold of medical indigency.

The threshold at the out-patient department and at admittance to the in-patient service in the New York municipal hospitals was set much more by pragmatic humanity than by econometrics. But the sort of person who insists on stricter criteria might find the underlying, supporting facts uncomfortable.

Let us try a little exercise in domestic arithmetic: If we spend more than 6 per cent of our national income on personal health services and if the national average expenditure now exceeds $200 per capita, then the $800 needed to buy medical care for a family of four requires an income of more than $15,000 before taxes if the expenditure for medical care is to be a fair charge to that family's income. Such an income is enjoyed by less than 10 per cent of this country's families. This is not to say that 90 per cent of the population is medically indigent, nor that many families realize they are medically indigent because they are not seeking the care they ought to be getting at all times. But it is fair to say that 90 per cent are at all times exposed to the hazard of medical indigency and can be reduced to general indigency by a sufficiently catastrophic medical experience.

For the population of New York the great Indian giver, Medicaid, has without doubt raised the threshold of medical indigency higher than it was before. A visitor to the municipal hospital emergency room was confronted with a bill—in 1969, for $11—in order to encourage his sign-up for means-testing by the Department of Welfare. No one insisted that the charge be paid then and there, but the bill itself sets up a serious psychological hurdle against the next return visit. The infant had better be really sick the next time to justify the anxiety and humiliation his mother has had to experience on this occasion. No such transaction blighted municipal medicine in New York City, for all its deficiencies, before Medicaid.

The Logistics of Medical Technology

The conclusion that the market cannot organize a technology as complex as medicine should come as no surprise to anyone who has a little familiarity with the U. S. industrial system. That system does not leave the organization and operation of any other high technology to the play of the market. The steel industry has integrated its technology from the mine to the warehouse and even to the final markets for a big portion of its total output. The same genius for logistics makes it possible for the auto industry to turn out ten million cars in one year. No one expects the American motorist to assemble his own automobile—to go to the warehouse to select this manufacturer's fenders, and that manufacturer's fins, and this set of headlights, and that motor, and so on. By the same token we cannot expect the consumer, medically indigent or not, to go out and organize the medical care he needs from the highly specialized working parts available to him here and there in the present system.

Reflections on this line led us, on the Commission on the Delivery of Personal Health Services, to our first recommendation to the City of New York: The city should get out of the hospital business. By this we meant that the city should abandon its frustrating and defeated effort to fill the gaps in the medical economy with its own inadequate facilities. I am sure that the same logic applies to every one of the giant county hospitals that stand in the middle of our larger cities—in Philadelphia, Chicago, Los Angeles. For every city government has had the same hobbles tied on its hands and feet by the brave reform administrations that have driven out the graft-ridden boss-dominated administrations from generation to generation. There is no evidence that the checks and balances that are supposed to keep officeholders honest in New York City prevent petty larceny; they seem, in fact, to encourage grand larceny in broad daylight. More important, the hobbles frustrate initiative and perpetuate incompetence.

It is impossible for the New York City government to manage a chain of hospitals. The Commissioner of Hospitals of the City of New York cannot delegate to the administrator of any one of his hospitals the authority that administrator needs to run his institution; the commissioner cannot do so because he himself is not entrusted with that authority. And he cannot get it from the Mayor because the Mayor does not have the authority either. The checks and balances system dissipates that authority among half a dozen overhead agencies within the city government and ties the rest to purse strings in Albany and in Washington, D.C.

The Commission on the Delivery of Personal Health Services recommended, therefore, that the city should try to secure the delivery of personal health services to the people by contract. The city, we said, should hire the private, voluntary institutions that command the resources of modern medicine to serve the public need. And we urged the city to turn its own hospitals and personal health service facilities over to a public-benefit, nonprofit Health Services Corporation in the private sector which would operate under contract to the city. The contract, as we envisioned it, could be the joint instrument of public authority and private initiative. By contract, the two parties could seek to bring about the rational structuring of the delivery system appropriate to the character of medical technology and responsive to public needs.

Flow charts and organization tables for the integration of the highly differentiated and specialized working parts of the technological apparatus of medicine have been on the drawing boards since the first Hill-Burton legislative hearings at the end of World War II. These idealized systems invariably place a medical school and its teaching hospital at their peak or center. With six medical schools and as many more first-rank teaching hospitals in New York City, there are more than enough resources in that city to give each borough its own regional health service system.

But the design of systems of this kind should turn on people and not on institutions and political jurisdictions. The system must be designed to place the individual consumer, the patient, at its center. From the moment he enters a doctor's office or any other site of primary care, he should be placed within the reach of whatever resources he requires.

The laissezfaire economy in medicine tells us very little about the relationship of resources to needs. There is now, for example, no reliable basis for saying how many physicians with this or that competence are required to serve a given unit of the urban population in our country. That is a question that ought to be of considerable interest to medical schools; it is one about which they are bound to learn more as they get into closer relationship with their communities.

If we can accept prevailing availabilities, however, it appears that about one thousand people will keep a physician employed and that thirty or fifty thousand will occupy the talents of the thirty or fifty physicians it takes to present the full competence of the medical specialties in a well-staffed ambulatory care center or a group-practice clinic. A population of a quarter of a million will keep a 500-bed hospital busy. Finally, a population of a million and a half to two million requires not only four or five 500-bed hospitals, but the full range of services that are to be found in a teaching hospital or medical school. In such a rationally structured system every ambulatory care center—every group-practice unit and every individual physician—would have ties to the community hospital; each community hospital in turn would be tied to the medical center of its region. Today, in the American system, informal channels of communication and referral already link institutions to one another and tie the smaller voluntary hospitals to the big medical centers.

Reconciling the Missions of Medicine
and Rationalizing Delivery

For the purpose of securing response to public need, however, these communities of affiliation must be made explicit and formalized by contract. One important objective would be to resolve the clash of missions—between service on the one hand and teaching and research on the other—that besets the medical schools. This is needed especially in New York, where the medical schools have taken on the responsibility for delivering medical services in the municipal hospitals. With the municipal hospitals once again the sink for patients rejected by the voluntary system, these medical schools are confronted with open-ended liabilities. In properly structured regional federations such liabilities would be equitably distributed to the participating institutions. Each community hospital would be obliged to receive and care for anyone in its community requiring its services. The medical school, in charge of the regional medical center and backstopping the community hospitals with its command of the full spectrum of medical technology, would carry a selective burden of service appropriate to its teaching and research mission. Each of the big medical centers in New York, however, is deciding that it must also function as the community hospital for its immediate community—because members of Students for a Democratic Society, having acquired bachelor's degrees, are now turning up in the medical schools and are insisting that the medicine they are learning be relevant to society.

What I have described here is another task for our universities in promoting the orderly evolution of our society. The universities, in fact, are the model of the third sector in the American social and economic order, the sector that stands between the governmental public sector, on the one hand, and the private sector, on the other. This third sector now produces nearly one-fifth of our gross national product and engages what is, by all odds, the principal intelligence of our population. Health services, in turn, present the model for the new relationship that is developing between the university and society. In projecting that relationship I am mindful of the need to defend the autonomy of the university if it is to serve as the source of rational alternatives at the crucial branching points in the evolution of our society.

A fully comprehensive health service system lays as much emphasis on preventive and supportive measures as on the treatment of illness and injury. Martin Cherkasky has described the object as narrowing the front door of the hospital and opening up the back door. The rising cost of medical care requires this rationalization of the precious resources of medicine. Some portion of the inflation in the medical economy can be charged to the upgrading of wage scales, which in the past have made nonprofessional hospital employees the principal involuntary philanthropists of American medicine. But most of the cost increases reflect the unconscionable waste of resources that is encouraged by the present modes of compensating and reimbursing physicians and institutions.

In a structured regional system it becomes possible to establish economic and social incentives for more efficient use of resources. It becomes possible, for example, to encourage alternatives to the fee-for-service system in the compensation of physicians. With more than a quarter of the physicians in the country (40 per cent in New York City) employed full-time on salary in medical schools and hospitals, full-time salaries are becoming fully competitive with the incomes that can be earned in private practice.

We have other models, such as the capitation payment of physicians, demonstrated in the Kaiser Health Plan in California and in the Health Insurance Plan in New York. Certainly some such alternative to fee-for-service must be developed to integrate the relationship of individual specialists and practitioners to the totality of service that they render as a group. No certified public accountant could possibly develop a rational analysis of the cost of individual inputs to the operation of, let us say, an intensive care unit.

In the economics of the Kaiser Health Plan one sees some of the advantages of a rational medical economy. In the Kaiser system it takes five hundred beds to serve a subscriber population of a quarter of a million. At the 1969 rate of prepayment by the client population, that represents an income of $25 million. Elsewhere in the country a typical 500-bed hospital operates as a $10 million business and goes broke. In the Kaiser setup it takes $10 of capital investment per head to render the services paid for at the rate of about $100 a year per head. The managers at that system can also tell us how many interns, pediatricians, obstetricians, and so on it takes to render good care per 10,000 population. No other source of intelligence in our medical economy can provide equally valid denominators for the planning of health care.

One might argue that the Kaiser experience represents the services required by a highly selective income-earning segment of our population and so does not represent the general experience of the whole. Let us double the cost—to equal the average annual expenditure by the population as a whole—and let us double or triple the investment in facilities. The Kaiser model still shows how the system can be structured and organized to deliver care of a quality not now available at costs exceeding $200 a head in our country.

The New Local-Centered Health Agency

From what I have already said, the role of public authority in the delivery of health services should be self-defining. As the contractor purchasing health services for the citizenry—and, in the process, supplying the major portion of the capital requirements and operating income of the health service system—the government has got to qualify itself to write and secure fulfillment of the health service contract. This cannot be done at the national level. The medical economy is a local one and medical services are rendered ultimately to the individual. So, city by city, we must see to the creation of an entirely new kind of health agency. In the governments of the cities we must establish health agencies charged with assignments not now covered by any public agency at any level in the government.

Monitoring Health Needs

The first of these assignments is to monitor the health needs of the population—to practice an entirely new kind of epidemiology that monitors the health of the population, assesses its needs, and fixes the denominators by which the distribution of resources is to be determined. In New York City, the health services administration would track the following sort of development: In two health districts in the South Bronx there was, in 1947, a population of 25,000, with 50 physicians in residence. In 1969, in those same two health districts, there was a population of 50,000 people—needless to say, its ethnic identity totally transformed—with 5 physicians in residence.

That development would be tracked and monitored by the city health agency. The early warning signals would go up and the facilities and services required to handle this enlarged and changed population would be installed to do the job.

Allocating Resources

The second assignment of the new city health agency is to plan the allocation of resources. Planning has been specified as a governmental function in both federal and state legislation. It is the decisive power in the framing and implementation of public policy; the responsibility for it must be plainly and unequivocally lodged with the government. A wise local government will, of course, share with the private sector the task of meeting that responsibility. But there must be no equivocation about the fact that planning is the responsibility of the elected officials and their appointed administrators.

Securing Public Accountability

The power and the ability to monitor needs and plan resource uses qualifies the city health service agency to fulfill its ultimate assignment, which is to secure public accountability of the institutions and persons rendering services under the public contract.

What I have described here is the need not only for a new kind of public agency, but for a new kind of public doctor, one who can find in the trends and movements of statistics the same kind of satisfaction that moves a young man to seek the face-to-face patient-physician relationship. The new ethical imperative has been described by C. H. Waddington: "The most powerful forces operating in the world with which we have to grapple intellectually and morally are directed toward such ends as changes in the statistical indices of infant mortality or nutrition. The idea of the good as we see it forcing the pace of historic change around us is not by any means only or even most importantly concerned with inter-individual reactions. It can hardly be expressed in any terms except those of statistical parameters."

Walsh McDermott sums it up by saying that we need "statistical compassion, a compassion for those we never get to see."

4

Perspectives on a Positive Manpower Policy

Garth L. Mangum

With the end of an innovative decade, it may be useful to examine what has been wrought in the matter of manpower—not that anybody started out to make a manpower policy. It simply emerged. In fact, I do not suppose we ever really make policies in a democracy. We attack particular problems that seem to have reached crisis proportions. Then we look back later and perhaps—if we are lucky—see some kind of coherence. This has been the process, a reaction to short-run phenomena—primarily in this case the high levels of persistent unemployment that accumulated around the late 1950's and early 1960's, followed by the transfer of interest in the civil rights movement from equal access to public facilities to getting a job so that money could be earned to make that access meaningful.

Some Long-Run Trends

There were long-run trends underlying the developments in employment. These basic, underlying trends are the four great imperatives of our age: technological change, urbanization, the coexistence of poverty and affluence—poverty amid affluence, rather than the traditional little bit of affluence amid poverty; and constant warfare. These are not independent phenomena. They are intermingled in a very complex way. They feed on each other: technological change, speeding urbanization, increasing affluence, but at the same time increasing the demands for preparation to participate in the labor market; urbanization and the consequent specialization, secularization, and rationalization that goes with it also contributing to increased affluence, but building in a kind of segregation that is extremely difficult to eradicate. It is a segregation based on economics rather than on actions which can be changed by changes in human intent. Both of these, again, contribute to affluence, which then leads to a situation in which, at least in our country, most are relatively well-to-do and therefore those who are not, feel relatively worse off than they might otherwise have felt.

And because of this basis in technological change and urbanization, more and more the individual's economic status is being determined by the formal preparation he has for participation in society. This in turn contributes to segregation on the basis of economic status—all these phenomena making for a built-in revolution of rising expectations in our own country.

Finally, war both speeds the rate of change and sops up the resources that might have been used to attack these problems. It also increases the inflationary cost of trying to do something about the manpower problem.

World War II and Its Aftermath

The beginning point of these long-run trends cannot be easily found. But we can look back to World War II and its immediate aftermath as a period in which there was an acceleration of the rates of change. We suddenly found ourselves with the task of feeding and arming much of the world, at a time when we had taken ten or eleven million of our prime-age labor force out of the production system, given them rifles, and sent them off to other activities. That required us to make some rather dramatic changes, and we did.

We accelerated the rate of rural-to-urban migration, pulled people out of rural areas and placed them in urban economic production. We took women out of the kitchen and put them into the labor force. We accelerated the pace of technological change, replacing men with machines. All of these developments turned out to be irreversible; our labor markets have never been the same since, nor has our society.

Then we capped all of that with the GI benefits law. In it we made a major social and economic decision for essentially noneconomic reasons. We said: "Here are a lot of people we want to reward for the years they've lost; in addition, we don't want them to re-enter the labor market too fast. Let's bribe them to stay out of the labor market and reward them by putting them in school." How many GIs went to school simply because $65 a month ($105 for those who were married) was offered for doing so? The 52-20 club wasn't going to last forever, so why not use those education stipends?

Education and Technology

A real social revolution resulted. People who would otherwise be driving trucks and working in mines now find themselves wearing white collars and doing very different things. Also altered were the trends in technological change. As we continued the technological acceleration that we had begun during the war, we could assume a relatively highly educated labor force. It is interesting to contrast our technology with that of Europe; the nations of Europe have a technology almost as sophisticated as ours but one which assumes far less technical education in the labor force.

Because we assumed a relatively well educated labor force, we built a technology that demanded it and caused increasing difficulty for those people who did not have that kind of formal preparation. That, in turn, fed on itself.

The new kind of migration, migration from rural to urban areas, was radically different from the old migration from foreign countries. There had been contiguity between the location of unskilled jobs and low-cost housing; in the postwar period that contiguity disappeared. Jobs increasingly moved out to the suburbs, following the more skilled and technically trained workers and the open spaces needed by the new technology in the factories. People were being located where housing economics and racial discrimination forced them to be, and that was a long way from the semiskilled jobs for which they were qualified.

Many other developments were hidden in the immediate postwar period by the demands to make up for wartime shortages followed by the Korean war. Then gradually during the 1950's, when relatively slow rates of growth caused employment to lag behind the acceleration in productivity and the more rapidly growing labor force, a new situation emerged, though it was not immediately obvious.

Since problems were identified by trial and error, it is not surprising that there were some misconceptions and some mis-starts. So the first assumption was this: Many people are unemployed, and where they used to be employed we now see machines working. Technological change must be the villain. Maybe the problem is that people do not have the skills that this technology requires. These people had substantial skills and played a significant role in the labor market in the past. Let's have a retraining program to make it possible for technologically displaced people to get back into the system.

But the slight resumption in the rate of economic growth soon pulled back into employment those people who had been technologically displaced. The problem was no longer the need for retraining programs; instead, the new retraining legislation had to become a training program for people who never had any skills in the first place.

As soon as that effort was undertaken, it was discovered that these people lacked basic educational skills, while all known training methods assumed that the trainee at least knew how to read, write, and figure. New remedial basic education was necessary.

These early programs assumed that most of the problems lay in the people; if you could change them, if you could give them skills and basic education, you could get them jobs.

Now we began to realize that there were not only problems of people, but that there were problems of the system. The people were either in depressed areas or in the central city ghettos, and the jobs were out in the burgeoning suburbs. People must be relocated from where they are to where the jobs are, or be able to commute. But transport had been built backwards: it was designed to bring suburbanites to their white-collar jobs, rather than to take central-city residents to suburban factories.

Start wrestling with that problem and you recognize that housing is very much intermingled with it. So is welfare. It is a tremendously complex series of forces that no one has yet been able to disentangle completely.

Wrestle with that problem and you discover that there are not enough jobs to go around. Maybe you have to create some jobs in depressed areas and ghettos. Maybe you are going to have to have public jobs as well as private jobs, so you experiment with a Neighborhood Youth Corps, with a work experience and training program, with a variety of other devices.

Tight Labor Markets and Hard-to-Place Workers

Then in the midst of all that the economy starts growing rapidly and you find yourself with a very tight labor market. Despite it, you still find yourself with a vast accumulation of unassimilated people in the labor market; the 1969 manpower report says there were 11 million workers who were jobless at some time in 1968. Even in the tightest labor markets we have ever had for any consistent period of time in all our history, and in the absence of wage and price controls, there are that many people who are simply not making out in the system. These are people who are still experiencing long-term unemployment. These are people who are looking for full-time jobs but can only find part-time ones.

These are people who for all observable reasons ought to be either working or looking for work, but who are not. Most interesting of all are the millions of people who work full time, all year, at wages which are not adequate to pull them up above the poverty level.

After wrestling with the problem of unemployment for six or seven years, it is suddenly the least important problem. What is to be done about underemployment and upgrading? People and jobs must be brought together. The subsidization of private employment appears to be worth some experiment. Out of that experience another piece of information, one we ought to have known but did not discover until recently, appears: those people in the central city ghettos are just as smart as anybody else. They act just like everybody else; when somebody offers them a job they ask whether the job is worth it, and they don't necessarily take any job that comes along. In tight labor markets there may be many jobs, perhaps even more jobs than people looking for jobs, but if the jobs are unattractive, if the pay is low, they may not be considered to be very important. The quality of a job may be more important than the quantity of jobs.

The most interesting single bit of information coming out of the National Alliance of Businessmen experience is the identification of the reservation rate in the urban ghettos, city by city, in over fifty cities. We now know that there will be no takers among young black males for a job that pays less than $2.00 an hour in Boston. In San Francisco the equivalent rate is $2.25. In San Antonio, if the offer is $1.60, there will be a stampede.

We begin to realize more about the way that system works and recognize that a lot of these experimental programs really have not been consistent with realities. There have been some interesting programs; some of them worked well, some not so well, but out of it all we have learned much. We now know that there are many people who need nothing more than skill training. With skill training they can get jobs. There are other people who need skill training plus remedial basic education. But both of these services are going to be useful and sufficient mainly for people who are already reasonably well motivated, people who are located where a job is within reach and who lack only the qualifications.

Beyond Skill Training and Remedial Education

There are people who need more, and people who are suffering the entire complex: lack of skills, lack of education, lack of locational access to jobs, lack of availability of a meaningful job worth taking in view of the individual's financial responsibilities and other opportunities for making an income.

We have gone through a long list of remedies, each one thought to be the ultimate panacea, each one supposedly providing *the* solution. Not long ago, it was felt strongly that the subsidization of private employers through the National Alliance of Businessmen program would do the job. A sense of disillusionment seems to permeate even the business community. It is a totally unjustified disillusionment. This program has really worked surprisingly well, but since it has not turned out to be as much of a problem-solver as it appeared initially, some of its champions are beginning to turn away from it.

Now we're moving on to other things; tax incentives, perhaps, or black capitalism. But one thing or another will always be *the* solution. If there is any one thing we ought to have learned over the last few years and have not, it is that there is no single solution. There are many partial solutions, each one of which will do some good for some people, but all one can do is continue to put together a more and more diversified package until one finally gets something that fits the whole group.

We have learned, for instance, that there is a variety of necessary services that we really never knew about before. We now know there is something called outreach. We do not use it; we do not have to, because the money and places are so limited that almost any program has more takers than it can support. But at least we know there is a population that we don't touch unless we get involved in outreach.

We know there is something called job development. We don't do much about it, though we have enough experience to know that it is not enough to expect people to adapt themselves to employers' job orders; we may also have to adapt the job to the people. Thus far job development has primarily meant pleading with the employer to take this client rather than someone else's client. But at least out of the experience we know that jobs must fit people as much as people must fit jobs.

The Vexing Problem of Evaluating
Needs and Programs to Meet Them

There has never been a time in the years since, perhaps, 1963 in which we have not had too much money to spend, given our capability to spend it wisely and the constraints attaching to the appropriations which forced us to spend it rapidly. Yet, paradoxically, we have never had enough money over a long period of time to have any meaningful impact.

We have never had an adequate way of measuring the extent of economic distress. We are still struggling along with a series of measures that were designed to measure resource utilization and that are badly adapted to measuring the degree of economic success. Experimentation with a universe-of-need concept is moving toward some measure of social distress.

We have never adequately evaluated any program, so we do not know what each has accomplished. This is hard to admit for one who has spent three years evaluating manpower programs, but it is true that we have never yet evaluated any manpower program with enough precision to say with any degree of assurance what it has or has not done. As a result, we have never been able to put the admininstrators' and program operators' feet to the fire and demand performance because we have no measure of performance.

We are only beginning to explore the appropriate relationship between federal, state, and local governments, and between national, regional, and community problems. Because programs have emerged with federal leadership—there was no other source of leadership—we created a series of programs that are expected to be nationally uniform. Every community is supposed to have the same combination of programs. Every community is expected to need so much institutional training and so much on-the-job training; so much work experience and so much basic education. There is no machinery to declare which community needs what combination of programs.

We have tended to do the same thing with individuals: We have a series of discrete programs and we say, "If you can fit within one of these programs, we'll do something for you." There is no machinery by which we can say, "Here is somebody who needs some skill training and some basic education, a set of false teeth, and relocation." We can't adapt a series of services to fit him.

Problems in the Delivery of Services

The problem of the delivery system has never been solved. Because we were concerned about the appropriate federal, state, and local relationship, we put together a cooperative area manpower planning system (CAMPS) hoping to build the capability at the community and the state level to do manpower planning. But we did not really trust the people at the state and local level. So we have issued them guidelines which say, "Here's exactly what you must do. We have drawn a set of boxes. You are to drop each of these numbers into the box that the 'feds' designate." We call that planning and have been surprised because people do not take it seriously. Recognizing, on the other hand, that there is no very good evidence that they would be capable of carrying out the responsibility if they had it, there is still a tremendous tendency (1) to ignore problems and (2) to attack the easy ones and let the more difficult ones go.

A concentrated employment program (CEP) was created. We were expecting every operator of an individual program to take that one program, hunt clients for himself, and force them into that program's mold. The least we should be able to do is put all the programs under one roof. Then we could at least open drawers and drop the people into the right program rather than make them fit the one available. But even that task is so complex that, given the administrative capability, few CEPs have ever worked as designed.

Then there is the whole issue of community action. There was a recognition that established agencies had picked clienteles who were more easily dealt with than some we had come to call the disadvantaged. There was a desire to create competitive institutions which could serve the poor and in which the poor could be represented. Experience has been that although these have been very effective as organizers of poor and demanders of service, by and large they have not been very good as deliverers of service.

Now we are in a quandary: If we give the delivery of service back to the established institutions, can these politically effective community action agencies stay alive? The realities of the political world are such that without patronage, without jobs and money to dispense, nobody pays much attention to you. If we take away the jobs and money which may not have been used very effectively, we may lose the value product, that which has been done rather effectively: organizing the poor and buying them into the political system.

There is the growing rebellion by mayors and governors. First mayors began to resent the fact that they had been bypassed in the manpower process. The tendency had been to go directly from the federal government to the ad hoc community groups. So the mayors demanded a piece of the action.

Then, in 1968, the governors began to recognize that not only had they been bypassed by the federal government going directly to the city level or to the community action organization; they were even bypassed when the federal government gave money to the states. The money and the power was going to autonomous state institutions—employment services and educational establishments that were, in most states, autonomous and independent of the governor. Now the governor wants his piece of the action.

Toward a Legislative Program Based on Experience

What finally emerges will be legislation of the following dimensions:

The attempt will be to take the budgets which now exist as individual programs, put them together, and make them available for a whole range of manpower services, rather than to continue earmarking particular chunks of money for particular services. Then a new relationship between the federal, state, and local governments can and will be pursued. The federal authorities have come to recognize that they cannot make all the wise decisions from Washington, as was once thought possible, but perhaps what they can do is provide a national perspective through guidelines, monitoring, and evaluation. They can say to state and local governments: "Here is money allocated to you for you to plan within these constraints. Here are the objectives. You come back and tell us how you plan to achieve them. We'll approve your plan and then you'll run the program." As a safeguard, a sizable amount can be kept back for national programs and for use in the recalcitrant states. Monitoring and evaluation can then reward the able and penalize the faulty in the next budget cycle. How far such legislation will get, time will tell.

There is growing interest in the kind of comprehensive manpower legislation which will route the money through politically elected officials (governors and mayors) who are responsible to some electorate. This may mean the end of a particularly interesting and quite fruitful experimentation in which we have done an unprecedented thing—that is, dump billions of dollars of federal money into the hands of institutions that were not responsible to any electorate or any group other than themselves. It also means the end of a trend taking social services out of politics. That has too often meant management by bureaucracies answerable only to themselves. Politicians are, at least, accountable.

There is also the issue in this learning process of who should work. In the December 1967 amendments to the Social Security Act, Congress decided that all those persons on public assistance capable of working had better work and whatever was necessary would be done to see to it that they work. The Work Incentive (WIN) experience has demonstrated that it is not so simple. The big decision to be made is whether mothers who are heads of families and have children work. If they should work rather than stay home and take care of their children, are we willing to provide the child care facilities and all the supportive services to make that possible?

An answer has not yet been necessary. The employment services, contrary to their expectations that they would be flooded with welfare recipients, have found themselves overmanned in the WIN program. The welfare administrators, having a somewhat different orientation, are not terribly anxious to submit their clients to the not-so-tender mercies of people who think that everybody really ought to get out and work.

Finally, in 1968, we faced the ultimate issue—the relationship between prevention and remedy. All the emphasis throughout the years has been on the tremendous backlog of underprepared, undereducated, mislocated people. Now, however, the recognition is growing that we are still dumping underprepared people into the labor market pool more rapidly than all of the remedial programs can siphon them off. Can we do a better job of preparing people for participation in urban labor markets in a day when the transition from school to work is becoming more difficult? Kids no longer have a way of gradually assimilating knowledge of the world of work. Some day they are going to be shoved or are going to jump out of school into the labor market pool, where they are going to splash around wildly, some to sink and others to learn to swim. The ones who learn to swim may find many opportunities, but we are becoming concerned lest we are losing too many of them.

Manpower Policy Achievements Viewed in Perspective

I have not painted the most sanguine picture in the world, I suppose. We really have not achieved any major solutions. Nevertheless, it has been a period of real accomplishment. Simply by attacking the problems, we have shown an increased sensitivity to human distress; that people in trouble are no longer docile but are demanding service is an additional accomplishment.

From a long-range viewpoint, we have been at the business of trying to build an effective school system for two hundred years and are still not completely satisfied with what we have. We have been experimenting with fiscal and monetary policies for at least thirty years, and still have a long way to go. In that perspective, the accomplishments of the years since 1962 in manpower have not been so bad.

In 1946 we made an important declaration of public policy in this country: the federal government would be responsible for seeing that adequate total supplies of economic opportunity are always available. We never did very much to fulfill that promise until recently; at the end of the 1960's we not only began to try to do something about the commitment of 1946, but went even further. We now admit that it is not enough to worry about the total supply of economic opportunity. We must concern ourselves with the distribution of opportunity. Now we are promising to see that every major group has access to the economic opportunity that our system seems to supply so well. We are moving rapidly toward the point of considering it to be our duty to see that every individual gets his reasonable and realistic access to employment opportunities.

In approaching that commitment, we have achieved some major accomplishments. We have a big investment and it is up to us to make sure the nation earns dividends on it.

Part 3   Providing for the Essentials

5   The American System of Social Security: Agenda for the 1970's

Eveline M. Burns

The American social security system is now a third of a century old, and there seems to be a general feeling that this is a good time for taking stock, since it is clear that many problems are still unsolved. It is also becoming fashionable to assert that economic and social conditions have changed so much since the 1930's when the main lines of policy were set, that we need new and different programs, better adapted to the conditions of today and tomorrow. I would like to consider this last assertion more closely.

Changes Since the 1930's

What really has changed since the 1930's? First, of course, there is the spectacular rise in productivity, which has increased GNP from $203.6 billion in 1929 (it fell as low as $141.5 billion in 1933) to $706.9 billion in 1968 (at uniform—1958—prices).[1] Even when allowance is made for the equally spectacular increase in population, income per capita has shown a remarkable rise. From the point of view of social security policy, this development might have been expected to have eased the task of the income-security policy-maker in several ways. First, it might have been expected that, with rising incomes, the numbers in poverty would have fallen and that the average income receiver, being better off, could now make more adequate provision from his own resources against occasional interruptions of income. Hence, the need for governmental action would presumably be less. Second, because of rising incomes, the possibility of providing everyone a minimum income without checking incentive would be greater. For the gap between the minimum and what could be secured by participating in production would

67

steadily increase, i.e., the "carrot" would be larger. Third, to the extent some public action was called for that involved a transfer of income from the richer to poorer, higher incomes would make it possible to raise taxes and still leave the average income receiver with an ever larger disposable income. Hence, the task of financing any given level of expenditures would be eased.

The last expectation has indeed been realized (average per capita disposable income having increased from $1,236 in 1929 to $2,473 in 1968, at uniform prices) although it seems likely that any further major increase in the tax take will meet considerable resistance.[2] But the first two advantages have not fully materialized. We have discovered that the gains of rising GNP have not been equally distributed and that there is still a disturbing amount of poverty. And at least to some extent, we have redefined in an upward direction the concept of the minimum level of income below which we classify people as being poor. Moreover, even at higher income levels people still seem to want to rely on public programs to assure incomes, at least in old age, as witness the pressure to raise the taxable income limit in OASDI to $12,000 or even $15,000.

A second obvious contrast with the 1930's is the lower level of unemployment. This, too, might have been expected to have reduced the need for government action, or at least to suggest different programs. But although the absolute numbers of the unemployed are very much less, unemployment is still a major hazard to security. In 1966 and 1967, both years of relatively low unemployment, some 5 million workers drew insurance benefits amounting to about $2 billion, and in more recent years beneficiaries have represented less than half, indeed nearer one third, of all the unemployed workers.[3] In 1966, nearly 11.5 million people experienced some unemployment, a fourth of them for 15 or more weeks. About a million were unemployed for more than six months.[4] Nor, I suggest, would we be wise to count on perpetuation of current low levels of unemployment. It is only seven years since 1961, when benefit payments rose to over $6 billion, and we cannot dismiss the possibility of future recessions. The character of the unemployed group has indeed changed, in that we now seem to have two major groups of workers: those who are more or less steadily attached to the labor market, often protected by seniority rules, who if dismissed are entitled to unemployment insurance benefits; and a second group, on whom are concentrated the brunt of employment fluctuations, if, indeed, they succeed in securing any attachment at all to the labor market. These are the older workers, the young entrants or potential entrants and the increasing group of educationally and socially disadvantaged workers from the rural areas and the South who are moving into the cities and the North. I doubt, however, whether conditions are very different from what they were in the 1930's. Then, too, we had especially heavy unemployment among older workers, and among the young, and the parents of the generation now seeking opportunity in the cities were suffering underemployment in the south and rural areas. The big difference is in visibility. As we cream off the favored groups protected through unemployment insurance, we become more aware of the common characteristics of the groups in which long-period unemployment is concentrated.

There is, indeed, one major difference between the 1960's and the 1930's. In the earlier period something was done about these types of unemployed. The Farm Security Administration programs assisted the rural poor. The Civilian Conservation Corps (CCC) and the two types of National Youth Administration (NYA) programs gave employment and/or training to large numbers of young unemployed. Between 1933 and 1940, over 2.25 million youth were enrolled in the CCC. The Out-of-School NYA program employed over 1 million youth between 1936 and 1940, and the NYA Student Work Program aided more than 1.5 million and young people between 1933 and 1940, almost half a million being on its rolls in April, 1940.[5] These figures make our current efforts to do something for the young unemployed look rather pitiful. And a sizable fraction of the adult long-period unemployed were given jobs through the Works Progress Administration (WPA), which between 1935 and 1940 gave employment to 7.8 million different people, the monthly numbers fluctuating between 1.45 million and 3.33 million.[6]

From the point of view of policy and program, I am suggesting that the main effect of lower levels of unemployment is on the sheer numbers for whom measures have to be planned, and that the nature and circumstances of the unemployed, knowledge about which should surely determine the policies to be adopted, are not so greatly different. In one way, however, rising levels of employment have made the task of the social security policy-maker difficult. For they have created an expectation that this should greatly decrease the need for public aid. As the number of public-assistance recipients has risen in recent years the program has come under increasing attack from those who believe that employment is the answer to personal insecurity and who fail to inform themselves about the characteristics of the public-assistance recipients. The prevalence of the belief that the recipients have only themselves to blame for being poor translates itself into pressure on policy-makers and administrators to be "tough" and illiberal in the assistance programs. Yet only a small fraction of the caseload consists of employable people. Of the 10.25 million assistance recipients in July 1969, 2.88 million were over 65 or disabled or blind, while another .75 million, mostly elderly or sick, were recipients of general assistance. The bulk of the load, 6.6 million, consists of broken families assisted through Aid to Families with Dependent Children (AFDC): 1.7 million adults and 4.9 million children.[7]

It is not easy to decide whether the sharply increasing number of dependent families is a "new fact," not present in the 1930's, of which we must take account in future planning. On the one hand, families headed by a woman have become a larger proportion of all families, although the high rate for nonwhites (23.7 per cent) has leveled off since 1959; and out-of-wedlock births per 1,000 unmarried women of childbearing age have tripled since 1940, although here, too, the rate has stabilized since 1959. But on the other hand, we do not know how many dependent broken families existed prior to AFDC, for we had no way of counting them. Only when, through enactment of AFDC, the nation undertook to provide income to such needy families and statistics began to accumulate did we discover with dismay how many there were.[8]

A third development bearing on social security planning is the impact of technological change. I do not share the gloomy forecasts of those who envisage a future with a constantly declining demand for labor and a need to ration work as a scarce and valuable opportunity and to provide income to the unemployed majority. Quite apart from the dubious political viability of such a society I cannot believe that the nation's demand for goods and services will be so easily satisfied, especially in the service area, which is least likely to be affected by automation. It is true there will be more need for tide-over income as people are retrained and relocated. But the great danger to the social security system, if we do find it desirable to change the balance between production of more goods and services and more leisure, is that there will be pressure to take the easy way out by concentrating access to more leisure on the aged through progressive lowering of the retirement age. This is pressure we should withstand. If there is to be more leisure, it should be distributed more equally among all age groups through changes in working hours, more holidays or sabbatical leaves, more vacations for housewives, and similar policies.[9] We should not let the social security system be perverted by forcing it to deal with problems more properly handled in other ways.

The big change that has taken place in the last 30 years has occurred in the area of social attitudes and values. First, there is now a greater acceptance of the role of government, and especially the federal government, in dealing with problems of economic insecurity. Despite the many programs developed in the early 1930's, they were all labelled "emergency measures" and expected to be short-lived. There was still great suspicion, if not fear, of governmental action and government itself had little experience in administering programs involving the distribution of cash benefits to individuals. All this has changed. Despite a lingering preference for private action over public (e.g., private business involvement in job-training or employment-opportunity programs, administration of Medicare by private intermediaries) and a general glorification of the private, as opposed to the public, sector there appears to be a conviction that major income security programs can only be effectively run by government and there seems to be much less reluctance to invoke governmental activity when the private sector appears unable to grapple with a social problem. I suspect that much of this changed attitude is due to the operational success of our major social security program itself, namely OASDI.

Second, there appears to be, if not a greater sensitivity to, at least an enforced widespread concern about, proverty, income insecurity and inequality of opportunity. This is likely to continue, thanks to the increasingly vocal and political pressure of the minority groups, including the millions now dependent on welfare, and it is supported by our rising affluence, which intensifies the contrast between the poor and the rest. We can no longer sweep these problems under the rug.

Third, there appears to be growing acceptance of the idea of a guaranteed minimum income for all, available under conditions that do not inhibit or destroy dignity and self-respect in the recipient. Advocacy of such a policy by a group of the nation's business leaders or through a manifesto from a thousand economists would have been inconceivable in the 1930's.[10] Here again, much of the credit, if such it be, for the change of public attitude must be given to our public social security programs over the past 30 years, which have accustomed us to the idea that giving people rights to benefits in stated contingencies does not spell the end of our free enterprise system.

Finally, there is a much greater tolerance of high tax levels than would have been thought possible before World War II. When the Committee on Economic Security framed the proposals which were in essence embodied in the Social Security Act of 1935, there was great concern about the expected public reaction to the taxes involved, especially as they meant taxing very low incomes for the first time. The maximum social security tax of 6 per cent was thought so provocative of shock that it was deemed wise to approach it by easy stages. Today we blithely contemplate a social security tax rising to 11.8 per cent, and this at a time when, profiling from what was learned from the collection of social security taxes, the Treasury now levies income taxes on the lower-income groups to help finance the other costly governmental services, including defense.

What I am saying is that I do not think there has been a great change in the nature of the basic problems which we try to deal with in our social security programs, although the numbers in certain risk groups may be larger or smaller than 30 years ago and we at least have the advantage of knowing rather more about the characteristics of the different groups, although not nearly as much as we should and could. The big changes have been in social attitudes, and all of them have been of a kind that increase our policy options. But before considering what new or changed policies we might envisage, one must ask what it is the American people want their social security programs to do.

The Objectives of Social Security

It seems to me social security has two major objectives, whose relative importance has changed from time to time. First is the elimination of poverty through provision of some minimum income. Second is assurance of the maintenance of some specified fraction of previous incomes in the event there should be an interruption or loss of earning power. To some extent the two objectives converge and are indistinguishable. It would, for instance, be difficult to say whether the spur to action in 1935 was a concern about widespread poverty due to the depression or a desire for income maintenance as the depression revealed that higher paid workers and even the middle classes were liable to suffer interruptions of earning power. Certainly, in the late 1920's the drive for old age pensions was pretty clearly motivated by a concern about poverty in old age. And equally certainly, many people are kept out of poverty by their income-maintenance payments, a fact which justifies applying the appellation "poverty preventive" to our social-insurance programs.[11] But after the passage of the Social Security Act the predominant emphasis, until recently, has been on income maintenance rather than poverty elimination. More attention has been paid to raising benefits at the upper income levels than to making sure that the minimum benefits are indeed adequate to provide a standard of living above the poverty line. And, again until recently, little attention has been paid to the effectiveness of public assistance payments in moving people out of poverty.

With the growing concern about poverty, however, it has become evident that the two objectives are not identical. An income-maintenance program aiming to guarantee some specified percentage of previous earnings cannot provide an above-poverty standard of living to workers whose full-time earnings were already below that level, even if the guarantee were 100 per cent, which it rarely is. Furthermore, interruption or loss of income, the concern of the income-maintenance programs, is not the only cause of poverty. Substandard earnings in full-time employment and family size and heavy charges on income, such as medical care, costs play an important role. On the other hand, a program whose clear aim is to guarantee some percentage of previous earnings cannot be criticized, as it is by some economists, for making some payments to people who are not poor.

The currently popular concept of "efficiency" would be relevant only if the single aim of the system were the abolition of poverty. But the American people appear to have two other concerns which policy makers must take note of. First is a concern about maintenance of initiative; specifically, willingness to work, to support oneself and one's family by earning, if this is possible. Second is a concern that, by and large, income guarantees or antipoverty payments be available under conditions that are not demeaning or destructive of human dignity and self-respect.

Work Incentives and the Need for Job Creation

The problem of incentive would occasion little difficulty if at least one of the three following conditions was satisfied: (1) if strong social pressure was exercised through religious sanctions or loss of valued status on those who did not behave in the socially approved manner; (2) if work was intrinsically fascinating, pleasant or satisfying to the performer or conferred high status; (3) if there was a strong desire for a standard of living higher than that assured through security payments, coupled with a realistic expectation that available jobs would indeed yield such a higher standard.

Contemporary society does not completely satisfy any one of these conditions. The force of religious sanctions and even of the Protestant ethic is clearly less powerful than it once was, especially among the very groups most directly involved, namely those whom poverty and deprivation have separated from the rest of society and largely alienated from its values. Much work is far from intrinsically interesting, and here again this is especially true of the kind of jobs likely to be available to the poverty and near-poverty groups. We have indeed succeeded marvelously in creating a widespread desire for more and more goods and services, and here our advertising institutions must be regarded as a real help to the social security policy planner. But although we are beginning to realize that much has to be done by way of equipping potential workers physically and educationally to fill available jobs, we have not made sure that enough jobs at rates of pay significantly higher than the poverty minimum are in fact available.

The big gap in our social security system is indeed in the area of job creation. Our first priority should be to round out the system with a program or series of programs assuring jobs at rates of pay above the poverty line. Such a policy would not necessarily mean the WPA kind of job, where government is the direct employer, although I suggest to you that we should take another look at what I still regard as the remarkable and imaginative achievements of WPA.[12] Governmentally stimulated job creation could also take the form of subsidies; either, as some political leaders now propose, to private industry or, as I believe to be more realistic and desirable, to organized social services, public or nonprofit, in the fields of health, education, social welfare, recreation, environmental beautification and modernization and the like, to facilitate the employment of additional personnel, the need for which has been amply demonstrated in all studies of our social service industries.

If we could inaugurate a policy that makes government the socially acceptable assurer of job availability (I hope we can think of some better concept or phrase than "employer of last resort," which sounds so funereal) we would have created conditions in which a reasonable man, inspired with truly American initiative but also concerned that his family not suffer because he is employed, would have a reasonable alternative to reliance solely on some publicly guaranteed income. The point is that in far too many cases this alternative does not now exist.

Obviously, jobs at some significant rate of pay above the poverty level would not solve the security problem of the large family, which, as we are increasingly realizing, is itself an important cause of poverty. But here the adoption of a children's allowance system, making payments universally, would help.[13] For with a significant children's allowance program in effect, the dollar amount of both the poverty minimum and the wage which would yield a plus above this could be lowered. For the minimum would then be set by reference to the needs of a man and wife only (or if the children's allowance was payable only for the second and subsequent child, on the basis of a man and wife and one child).

A public program for making jobs available must be seen as an indispensable complement to our existing security programs. Quite apart from the fact that it would minimize the cases in which the desire to work is currently thwarted by the nonavailability of jobs paying more than the poverty equivalent, it would make more effective such controls as the requirement that able-bodied adults register at employment offices (and face disqualification for refusal to accept suitable work). It would also serve as a substitute for minimum-wage legislation, as the experience of WPA showed.

Incentive Provisions in Social Security Programs

We are putting an intolerable, indeed an impossible, burden on our social security programs by requiring them to deal with the problem of incentives. The effect is particularly unfortunate in regard to the programs that frankly aim at the removal of poverty; namely, public assistance and the currently fashionable Negative Income Tax (NIT). Both programs embody the same policy: to make up the difference between the income people have and what they should have if they were to be brought up to at least the minimum that would remove them from poverty. The difference between them lies in the fact that the NIT is a federal program (although this would disappear if the proposal of former Secretary of Health, Education and Welfare Wilbur Cohen and others for a federalization of public assistance were adopted); it uses the tax authorities rather than the welfare agency as the administrator; it adopts an income declaration rather than an exhaustive individualized investigation of all resources and a standard payment in place of an individualized calculation of a family's needs; and finally, it applies to the working as well as the nonworking poor. Yet, in some states even this difference is very slight. In New York State, with its increasingly simplified payment standards, its adoption of the income declaration or affidavit in place of the detailed investigation of resources, its limitation of mutual family responsibility to the nuclear family, and its willingness to supplement wages, the program is increasingly indistinguishable from the NIT in all essential particulars.

Both public assistance and NIT find themselves involved in the incentive problem. Both place their faith in the same solution. To avoid discouraging the recipient from working, they would allow him to retain some portion of his earnings without jeopardizing his claim to a public payment. In public assistance terminology, one disregards some fraction of an applicant's earnings in assessing the resources that have to be set against his needs as determined. In NIT one taxes earnings at less than 100 per cent.

But both programs are finding that if "notch" problems are to be avoided, payments must be made to people who are above the poverty line; and the higher the poverty line or the smaller the tax on earnings, the higher will be the income of those entitled to some payment. Thus, one of the advantages claimed for both gap-filling programs, namely efficiency in not making payments to the nonpoor, begins to disappear.[14] The NIT proponents have reacted to this dilemma by proposing to fill only part of the poverty gap, thus passing the buck to the public assistance system.[15] Most public assistance systems have never aimed to fill the entire gap and have only recently begun to try to build in incentives by the policy of disregarding some fraction of earnings; but as they do so, they too will face the same dilemma.

This effort to build incentives into the payment system greatly complicates administration, especially when it is recalled that for many of the poverty group income is highly fluctuating and highly unpredictable. Finally, we still do not know much about the incentive effect of different rates of taxation on the desire to work.[16]

The Case for the Demogrant, or National Dividend

It is for these reasons that I question in principle the desirability of trying to build incentive devices into our income security programs, sad though this would be for economists who are having such fun today playing with models and formulae. Why do we not separate the system for making antipoverty payments from the system which determines how much of total received income people should return to their government in the form of taxes? After all, we seem to assume that those who are above the poverty line can be trusted to behave rationally in apportioning their time between work and leisure although they know that some part of their earnings will be taken by the government. Why not extend the same assumption to those below the poverty line, especially if, as I have suggested, there be made available jobs paying more than the poverty minimum?

Instead of public assistance, even if federally operated, or of the NIT, which would involve the confusion of adopting two definitions of income (one for NIT and one for tax collection purposes), why not pay everyone a demogrant, or national dividend, and let an individual earn as much or as little as he wishes and at the end of the year provide for a reckoning with government through the income tax system? This would enable us to make much more effective use of our tax system as the instrument for determining, in the light of all considerations and taking all incomes into account, how much of their income people should devote to the support of all our public services (including defense). In such a tax system, all income, including publicly provided income, would in principle be liable to tax, although it would probably be decided that, as now, incomes below a certain level would be immune from taxation.

Such a program will, of course, be objected to on the grounds that it would be impossibly costly. In fact, the net cost would depend on the tax policy, which would determine how much would be recouped from those above the poverty line. It would indeed involve a considerable measure of income redistribution, but this is inevitable if poverty is to be eliminated. It can also be admitted that under a universal demogrant, some people would be content to live on the minimum guarantee. In a program dealing with millions (for the group "at risk" would include not only those currently in poverty but also those who keep themselves above that line by a combination of work and some socially provided income), we will have to accept some degree of incentive loss as the price for having a system that does not penalize the many by onerous or unpleasant requirements in order to control the few. Are we not rich enough to pay this price? The question is, How large is the group likely to be if jobs paying significantly more than the poverty minimum are available?

For one population group, namely female-headed families, the problem of incentives presents peculiar difficulties. Should public policy encourage the AFDC mothers to accept employment if well-paying jobs are available for them (which of course they are not)? It is partly a question of how far society is prepared to make the extra investment in day-care and homemaker services that alone will enable many husbandless mothers to hold paid jobs without sacrificing the welfare of their children. It is partly a question of how far society is prepared to force low-income mothers with no husband in the home to carry the burden of two jobs—the one she is paid for and the one awaiting her when she returns home to her family. But ambivalence of policy will persist until we recognize that when we talk about the importance of work, we always mean work for pay. Thus, we place no value on the work a woman performs when caring for her own husband or children, but if she cares for other people's husbands and children for pay, then she is working. Failing the adoption of a universal demogrant, the possibility of a housewife's allowance is worthy of exploration.

In any case, even if we are unwilling, as yet, to provide for a demogrant covering the employable population, we could at least introduce it for the aged and the disabled (a subject to which I shall return) and for children.

The Desire for a System Without Degrading Conditions

Hitherto the objective of a system without degrading conditions has been achieved through the adoption of the social insurance technique. Benefits are payable as a right, subject to fulfillment of objectively determinable conditions that minimize the exercise of official discretion (primarily past labor market participation), because contributions have been paid by or on behalf of the worker, and the system can thus be likened to insurance, a respected institution. We still do not make as full use of this device as we could; far too many workers are excluded from coverage, especially in unemployment insurance, and it has not been applied to all risks, notably temporary disability, for which it would be appropriate. Indeed, I am not convinced that even the idea of insuring children against family breakdown should be dismissed out of hand. Filling these gaps is one of the more obvious items on tomorrow's agenda.

But the insurance systems have troubles of their own. Failing the availability of more appropriate and acceptable alternative programs, there has been pressure to expand the role of the social insurances to cover groups whose labor market attachment is extremely marginal; to pay unemployment benefits for periods longer than would seem desirable; and as more irregularly employed or low-paid workers are covered, to increase minimum benefits and push the system toward undertaking poverty-removal functions, as well as income maintenance. In consequence, the insured population can be expected to become restive at having to pay insurance contributions a substantial part of which go to paying for unearned benefits, and the social desirability of assessing the costs of these minimum guarantees on lower incomes is increasingly challenged.

More recently, the viability of the social insurance system faces a threat from developments in the poverty-removal programs. For as public assistance is liberalized, as emphasis is placed on legal entitlements, as administration becomes less offensive to the recipient, as affidavits replace detailed investigation and minimum payment standards are enforced, the line between assistance and insurance will become blurred. Lower-paid workers, in particular, may well wonder whether it is worth while paying social security contributions for the privilege of receiving a benefit that differs in few respects from the payments under poverty-removal programs. This question would become insistent were NIT to be enacted.

I have long argued that the only answer is not to try to combine in one way the same program the two social security objectives, guaranteeing a minimum above-poverty income and replacing a fraction of previous earnings, and I am glad to see that this view has also been adopted in the recent Brookings volume on Social Security.[17] But whereas the authors would provide for the poverty-removal objective by NIT, I would use a demogrant.

Implications for Existing Programs

Especially for the aged and the disabled, it should be possible even now to develop a double-decker system, as in Canada and some other countries, where there is a basic uniform payment, financed from the general revenues, to all who are above a certain age or who are certified as disabled, in addition to which workers would receive some fraction of their preretirement income in return for contributions. The big problem is how to make the transition. We might introduce the demogrant by degrees, as was done in New Zealand, providing for it to rise annually as national income rises and meanwhile holding down liberalizations, including increases of the minimum benefits, in the contributory social insurance system.[18]

Such a separation would have many advantages. It would free the contributory system of responsibility for financing unearned minimally adequate benefits. It would provide an appropriate place for the government contribution, which all now seem to agree will be necessary if we continue to use OASDI for both security objectives. It would ease the retirement test problem by making it possible to pay contributory benefits at a stated age with no earnings limitations and allow society to adjust the age of payment of the demogrant to the labor market needs of the economy. Above all, if relieved of the necessity to assure a basic minimum to all, the contributory system would avoid problems of income redistribution within the system. Used solely to finance deferred income, to replace some fraction of lost earnings, the social insurance contribution would indeed be a contribution and not a tax. It would be a planned deferment of take-home pay and, being an addition to the basic demogrant, could be determined by the relative values attached to present, as against future, income.

In unemployment insurance these advantages would not be reaped if it was felt unwise to provide a demogrant for the employable population. But if this was done, it would simplify the administrative task. Freed from the pressure to pay minimally adequate benefits to workers whose labor market attachment may indeed have been minimal, the system would not be burdened with the problem of maintaining incentives. The only problem would then be to test the extent of labor market attachment and level of earnings, which would automatically be answered by the wage record; and the involuntary character of unemployment, through use of the requirement to register at an employment office and face disallowance if suitable work is refused. Furthermore, if the unemployment insurance system were seen solely as a system for replacing some specified fraction of previous earnings, low or high, the problem of the treatment of the married woman worker would be eased. For the system would then not have to be concerned with the question of why women work or whether they are primary earners. They would be unemployed workers, entitled to payments whose amount would reflect their previous earnings.

Even in the absence of a demogrant applicable also to the employable population, some policies could be indicated. More strenuous efforts should be made to limit the coverage of the program to workers who have a substantial attachment to the labor market. The duration of benefits should not be extended beyond a period reasonably reflective of nonrecession, nonstructural unemployment. The present 26-week period seems adequate to cover most short-period labor market adjustments, including seasonal unemployment. Since we have, presumably, to accept a continuation of state, rather than federal, unemployment insurance programs, it makes sense to limit the functions of the programs to dealing with income loss due to short-period unemployment and unemployment of the type that does not lie outside the control of individual states. But recessional or structural unemployment, roughly measured by duration of unemployment, should surely be a federal responsibility. The type of program or provision called for involves more than just the payment of a benefit that has been devised to deal with short-period unemployment and to provide for nondeferable expenditures—which become increasingly nondeferrable as unemployment persists. Higher benefits, retraining and work programs are indicated, and these should be a federal responsibility.

No nondiscriminatory system providing specified benefits to specified persons in specified contingencies can cover all cases of need or emergency. Room has to be left in the system for a discretionary program, although one would hope its role would be small. Nor is it realistic to expect that a universal poverty-removing demogrant will be speedily enacted; and the best that NIT advocates appear to hope for is introduction of a system that goes only part way toward the abolition of poverty. Like it or not, the institution variously called the Poor Law, public assistance, public welfare, or social assistance still will have a role to play—relatively large now, hopefully minor and residual in the future. Our enthusiasm for new programs should not tempt us to relax pressure for the renewal of the public assistance program.

The objectives would be flat grants, as far as possible subject to federal minimum standards; need as the essential criteria for eligibility, to be tested by declaration and spot checks; and sympathetic administration of the discretionary elements. All this will involve a greater federal role in program financing and administration.

Conclusion

Those to whom the words "social security" are synonymous with "social insurance" will have wondered why I have devoted so much attention to the noninsurance programs. The emphasis has been deliberate, for the experience of our own and other countries has shown that the entire field of income insecurity is a single system. Efforts to develop a program that deals with only one part of the problem can never be really successful unless the other parts, too, are dealt with in appropriate ways. In the absence of acceptable and effective provisions for the other problem areas, there will be pressure on the preferred program to expand its responsibilities beyond the purposes for which it was initially devised, with the result that it can no longer attain its own objectives.

It is for this reason that as we plan for the future, we should follow certain policies:

1. The difference between the two demands which Americans make of their social security system must be recognized. The demand for assurance of some fraction of previous earnings in the event of inability to earn is not the same as the demand for assurance of some guarantee of minimum income which will be adequate to remove people from poverty. We should not try to attain both objectives in a single program.

2. We should not try to build into our cash-payment programs devices to avoid work disincentives. The system of making cash payments to people should be separated from the system which determines how much of their income, privately and publicly obtained, people should be allowed to keep for free disposal.

3. We must complete our income-security provisions by government action to assure the availability of jobs that pay more than the minimum guaranteed poverty-removing income, and this must be regarded as an indispensable part of the total social security system.

4. The most desirable method of assuring incomes that will move people out of poverty is the use of the demogrant, not the NIT or a federally administered or regulated public assistance system. The level of the demogrant would have to be determined in the light of productivity levels and other considerations. It should, however, be noted that the more certain elements in family expenditures are taken care of in other ways (e.g., health insurance or a free public health system, housing subsidies), the lower the

demogrant would have to be. And the question of whether the payment should be nationally uniform or subject to geographical differentials is one that will arise not only in relation to a demogrant but also in contemplation of NIT or a federally administered or standardized public assistance program.

5. A children's allowance is a necessary addition to the social security system. It would greatly ease the task of the social security planner, as well as making a sizable contribution toward the reduction of childhood poverty.

6. The OASDI program should be buttressed by the payment of a demogrant, financed from general revenues and payable to all the aged and disabled, with the insurance benefits being seen as a replacement of some fraction of previous income over and above the demogrant.

7. As long as we have no demogrant for the employables, the best we can hope for in unemployment insurance systems, apart from coverage extensions, is to restrict the scope of the state unemployment insurance systems to dealing with short-period unemployment, leaving to the federal government responsibility for providing for the long-period unemployed and the never-employed employable people, for whom the mere continuation of a specified fraction of previous earnings is not an appropriate provision. But it must be recognized that this will still leave the state unemployment insurance programs plagued by pressures to include people for whom an income-maintenance program is an inappropriate type of payment and to modify the system so as to provide not only for replacement of some fraction of lost income but also for an acceptable minimum benefit.

8. There will always be a role for a discretionary needs-based program within the total system. I am not so naive as to suppose that we shall immediately move to a system of social security that would be rational and comprehensive. Yet, I believe it important that we have in our minds the general direction in which we want to move, so that we may have some criteria against which to measure proposals and amendments. It is with this objective in mind that I have ventured to make the above general propositions.

Notes

1. *Economic Report of the President, January, 1969* (Washington, D.C.: U.S. Govt. Printing Office, 1969), p. 228.

2. Ibid, p. 245.

3. *Unemployment and Income Security: Goals for the 1970's* (Kalamazoo, Mich.: Upjohn Institute, 1969), pp. 11 and 13.

4. U.S. Department of Labor, *Work Experience of the Population in 1966,* Bureau of Labor Statistics Special Labor Force Report No. 91.

5. National Resources Planning Board, *Security, Work and Relief Policies* (Washington, D.C.: U.S. Government Printing Office, 1942), pp. 261, 265, and 270.

82 Social Economics for the 1970's

6. Ibid, p. 234.

7. *Social Security Bulletin,* November, 1969, p. 2.

8. There is considerable difference of opinion among welfare experts as to the possible existence of a new factor, namely "fiscal abandonment," whereby the father ostensibly "deserts" the family to maximize its total income from his own earnings plus the appropriate welfare payment for the "deserted" family.

9. Eveline M. Burns, "Income Maintenance Policies and Early Retirement," in Juanita Kreps, ed., *Technology, Manpower and Retirement Policy* (Cleveland and New York: World Publishing Company, 1966), pp. 125-240.

10. See, for example, the "report from the steering committee of the Arden House Conference on Public Welfare (a group of business leaders appointed by Governor Rockefeller) and "Statement by Economists on Income Guarantees and Supplements," both reprinted in Volume II of *Income Maintenance Programs,* Hearings before the Sub-Committee on Fiscal Policy of the Joint Economic Committee, U.S. Cong., 2nd Sess., June 1968. See also the report of the Heineman Commission.

11. Lampman estimates that 8½ per cent of all families in 1961 were kept out or taken out of poverty and received 28 per cent of all income transfers: Robert J. Lampman, "How much does the American System of Transfers benefit the poor?" in Leonard H. Goodman, ed., *Economic Progress and Social Welfare,* National Conference on Social Welfare (New York: Columbia University Press, 1966), p. 135. Merriam reports that in 1968, 6.8 million aged beneficiaries were kept out of poverty by their social security benefits: Ida C. Merriam, "Income Maintenance: Social Insurance and Public Assistance," in Shirley Jenkins, ed., *Social Security in International Perspective* (New York: Columbia University Press, 1969), p. 77.

12. For a brief account of the work programs of the 1930's see Security Work and Relief Policies, Chapter IX.

13. Eveline M. Burns, ed., *Children's Allowance and the Economic Welfare of Children, The Report of a Conference* (New York: Citizen's Committee for Children of New York, 1968); James C. Vadakin, *Children, Poverty and Family Allowances* (New York: Basic Books, 1968); and Alvin L. Schour, *Poor Kids* (New York: Basic Books, 1966).

14. The Heineman Commission has estimated that a negative income tax with appropriate incentive features and making payments up to the current poverty level would involve some payments to 24 million families. Far too little attention has hitherto been directed to the psychological and political consequences of making supplementary payments to so large a fraction of the population.

15. Thus, President Nixon's Family Assistance Plan would guarantee income only up to $1,600 annually for a family of four, and the more liberal Heineman proposal would guarantee only $2,400. Similarly, the proposals of Pechman, Tobin, Friedman, and other economists all fall below the current poverty level.

16. It is interesting, for instance, that a recent study of the OASDI retirement test on workers' earnings found that the effect of beneficiaries did not noticably differentiate between the $1 for $2 and the $1 for $1 reduction provisions in determining their postretirement earnings. Kenneth G. Sander, *The Retirement Test: Some Preliminary Findings Regarding Its Effect on Older Workers' Earnings,* Research and Statistics, Note 8 (Washington, D.C.: Office of Research and Statistics, S.S.A. Department of Health, Education and Welfare, May 1968).

17. Joseph J. Pechman, Henry J. Aaron, and Michael K. Taussig, *Social Security: Perspectives for Reform,* The Brookings Institution, Washington, D.C. 1968.

18. Burns, "Income Maintenance Policies and Early Retirement."

Comment

Henry H. Chase

Any attempt to represent the viewpoint of business is at best difficult and often impossible since the business community does not always share a uniform point of view. However, with respect to much of the subject matter covered in Dr. Burns' paper, it might be possible to present a business consensus. On many points, the reaction would be negative, but I am reasonably sure this would not be true with respect to the fundamental issues.

There is genuine concern at management levels with those sociological and economic problems that have come to the fore in the last few years. Comprehensive and in depth examinations are being made of such concepts as the negative income tax, demogrants, federal standards for public assistance—all kinds of proposals—to which management might have been expected to give little attention until relatively recently. This is not to suggest that there is necessarily going to be a sharp reversal in what you probably recognize as the prevailing, traditional business viewpoint. I am suggesting only that such concepts are being examined carefully and that the possibility of somewhat different viewpoints emerging should not be ruled out.

Some Basic Reservations

Dr. Burns raised two points that I particularly want to note. The first is her comment that the primary need—or as she refers to it, the big gap—in the social security system is for government to assure jobs at rates of pay above the poverty line. The second is her proposal—not a new one, of course, as she advocated it for many years—of a universal demogrant, or guaranteed minimum income.

Both concepts cause serious concern in business circles and give rise to a number of questions. The first and most obvious is that either of her proposals would cost a great deal of money. Second, there is considerable concern among businessmen, which Dr. Burns indicates the American public and apparently she herself share to some degree, about incentives.

Third, proposals of the nature referred to involve separating particular groups from the rest of society. If adopted, they would tend to pinpoint and further isolate groups that are in but not of our society. This possibility is a matter of deep concern to businessmen as they examine and attempt to evaluate proposed solutions for the elimination or alleviation of poverty. There is widespread feeling in the business community that they would be divisive and would tend to exacerbate existing differences between those who are economically self-supporting and those who are not. Obviously this is something we do not need a great deal more of in our society today.

There also seems to be a rather casual dismissal of the insurance concept, the concept of earned benefits or earned rights. To the business community, this concept is of real importance. Not only does it make a difference to the individual who is receiving payment, but also, and of equal importance, it makes a difference in the way others in the community view those who are receiving payment and in the way both those who are and those who are not being benefited view the payment. These views have been held in common, and over a long period of time, by many individuals whose viewpoints on other issues frequently conflict. Lately, however, they appear to have been ignored.

The Concept of Full Participation

Dr. Burns suggests that the biggest change that has occurred in this country in the last 30 years has been in the area of social attitudes and values. I agree with her. However, she cites as her prime example the fact that there has been a greater acceptance of the role of government, especially the federal government, in dealings with problems of economic insecurity. I am not sure I agree with that. It seems to me there has been a much more fundamental shift in the area of social attitudes and values. In my opinion, this has been the growth of the view that no group in this country should be shut out or set apart or denied the opportunity to participate fully in our society. Accordingly, whatever the solution may be to the really fundamental problem to which Dr. Burns' paper seems to me to relate, one thing seems certain: the solution can't be a "buy-out." The creation of a superwelfare program, by whatever term it may be called, simply does not appear to be a viable answer.

I have no plan developed or sponsored by management to resolve the problem. Management neither has nor claims to have a panacea. If the number of those in poverty continues to diminish as rapidly as it has during the last few years, it seems fair to say that the business community's expectation is that the basic solution will come largely as a result of employment in the private sector—at least for those who are employable or who can become so with proper training. In this connection, business feels that considerably more emphasis needs to be placed on those who, with help, can become self-supporting. If this is done, and if the new economics does, in fact, provide the road to a continually expanding economy, presumably the continued reduction in the number of those in poverty should proceed at an accelerating rate.

I am drawing a line between those who can rise out of poverty, if given the necessary opportunity, support, and help, and those who cannot. There is no assertion that every unemployed adult is able to enter the labor market or is capable of being trained to do so. It is not even maintained that it is appropriate that all of them should. Under the most ideal circumstances conceivable, there will be individuals who will require and who should have society's help in the form of direct financial support; however, a systematic attack on the causes of poverty and public dependency must be based on education and training for employment, and active participation in the labor market.

In this respect, Dr. Burns' view that a great deal has been done to equip the disadvantaged to enter the labor market and compete successfully is rather surprising. The prevailing business viewpoint is that while something has been accomplished in this area, very much more needs to be done. Far more emphasis has yet to be placed on basic education, training, and exposure to productive employment. Far more people need to be brought into the labor market and afforded the opportunity to become self-supporting.

The Role of the Private Sector

During the period when Robert Kennedy was seeking the Democratic nomination for the presidency, he expressed rather forcefully the viewpoint that the real need was to find a means of bringing more of the disadvantaged fully into our society and he related this directly to their participation in the private sector of the economy. In my opinion, business shares that view. The basic need is to make it possible for those who can work to do so, and by so doing enable them to become full-fledged members of society. The disadvantaged should not be compelled to live or, perhaps more accurately, to exist as appendages to society.

Dr. Burns says,

> Despite a lingering preference for private action over public (e.g., private business involvement in job training or employment-opportunity programs, administration of Medicare by private intermediaries, etc.) and a general glorification of the private as opposed to the public sector, there appears to be a conviction that major income security programs can only be effectively run by government and there seems to be little reluctance to invoke governmental activity when the private sector appears unable to grapple with a social problem.

To me it would seem that spokesmen in both major political parties, as well as a number of prominent individuals outside of politics, seem to be turning to the private sector, rather than to government, for solutions. Accordingly, I wonder if there is increasing, rather than diminishing, reliance being placed on the private sector to provide avenues by which the problem of poverty can be successfully attacked.

The points I have attempted to cover seem to me to be of greater significance than some of the specifics incorporated in Dr. Burns's paper, for example, children's allowances.

Elimination of Poverty as a Goal of Social Security

A statement of Dr. Burns's I would like to comment on relates to the development of the social security program, or perhaps more accurately to the character of that program. She stated that social security has two major objectives: the first is to eliminate poverty and the second is to deal with the problem of income interruption. I question whether there actually have been two major objectives and, further, whether even today there is general acceptance of the first objective she cites. Dr. Burns herself, after listing those two objectives, goes on to say that since the enactment of the social security program, the thrust has been to deal with the problem of income interruption. Until relatively recently, the early to mid 1960's say, there was little, if any, consideration given to the concept of lifting individuals out of poverty—at least as the term "poverty" is used currently. While this concept of a dual objective has appeared in recent papers—for example, the Brookings Institution publication *Social Security—Perspectives for Reform,* it seems to be a relatively recent discovery.

Certainly, the prevailing business viewpoint is that social security has not had and should not have as an objective the elimination of poverty. It is, of course, true that many individuals have been lifted out of poverty as a result of the benefits paid under the social security program. Merely because this has been a frequent result, it does not necessarily follow that it either has been or should be an avowed objective. It is evident that a number of fundamental issues arise if one accepts the assertion that the social security program has as its primary objective the lifting of people above the poverty level. As Dr. Burns suggests, considerable restructuring of the program would be required were we to attempt to secure that result. Indeed, If I understand her correctly, she says that the program does not really lend itself to that objective.

Labor's Reaction

Certain statements of Dr. Burns's are intriguing to me primarily because I am interested in labor's reaction to them. Dr. Burns says that if there is more leisure to be distributed, it should be distributed equally; that it ought not all be given to the aged; that is, the retirement age should not be lowered. At another point, it is suggested that a public program making jobs available would serve as a substitute for minimum-wage legislation.

Finally, she states that the social security tax was approached in small steps rather than by the immediate imposition of a 6 per cent levy because such a tax would have been shocking to people in 1935. I submit it would be rather shocking today if it were seriously recommended that the existing social security tax rate be increased by 6 percentage points. I suspect that shock would be expressed as much by labor as by the business community and the self-employed.

Comment

Bert Seidman

Dr. Burns concludes her provocative agenda for social security by pointing out that efforts to develop a program that deals with only one part of the problem can never be really successful unless the other parts too are dealt with in appropriate ways. This realization, I think, should guide all of our efforts to develop social welfare programs. Unless we recognize that we have a multifaceted problem, or, to put it another way, that we have many problems to deal with, we will not be able to achieve any of our objectives.

Changes in Social Attitudes and Values:
Many-Sided Problem

Henry Chase and I, starting from very different premises, I think, arrive at the same conclusion: that in stating the changes that have occurred in what Dr. Burns calls the area of social attitudes and values, she has been much too sanguine and optimistic.

First of all, she says there is a greater acceptance of the role of government. I agree that there is a greater acceptance of the role of government, but by no means do I think it has reached a very high stage as yet. I wish it had reached a much higher stage than it has.

Secondly, she says there is a greater sensitivity and concern about poverty. I think, again, that this is true. I am reminded of a meeting of the Washington chapter of the Industrial Relations Research Association I attended some years ago. Hyman Bookbinder, who later became Assistant Administrator of the OEO and was very active in the early stages of the poverty program, was the speaker. In the discussion I said that one of the things that distinguished the early 1960's from the 1930's was that during the earlier period people admitted the existence of poverty. Now I think it is very much to the credit of our country, and particularly to the credit of President Johnson and his administration, to have brought us back to an awareness and an acknowledgment of the existence of poverty. I would even say that we make this acknowledgment much more freely than many of the European countries (at least in the years that I was there); in the face of a great deal of poverty, they used to claim that they had eliminated poverty by what we would call the "new economics," yet we do not acknowledge poverty to anything like its full extent.

Thirdly, Dr. Burns says that there appears to be a growing acceptance of the idea of a guaranteed minimum income for all, and she contrasts this with the situation of the 1930's. I think I would say just the opposite; I would say that in the 1930's, because so many people were out of work, unemployed, and did not have an income, there began to be an acceptance (which did not last very long) that there should be at least some level of guaranteed minimum income for everyone. We did in fact have large-scale programs with this objective. We do have a growing acceptance of the idea now, but again I think it is not nearly as great as Dr. Burns seems to think—judging from the emphasis she has put on this point.

What I am really saying is that we do not have the degree of public support for the kind and degree of government intervention that seems to be implicit not only in Dr. Burns's analysis, but, even more important, in her policy prescriptions. Thus, arriving at it from a different direction, I agree with what Henry Chase says.

On the other hand, at a recent meeting in New York of the Committee for Economic Development, I did not hear one businessman of the two hundred or so in attendance get up to declare that the poor are just loafers. I presume those at the meeting were somewhat more liberal than average businessmen; they had assembled for a full day of discussion on public welfare and related questions—not social insurance, but public welfare. What they did say was along these lines: "I don't quite understand what this guaranteed annual income is, but whatever it is we have to do something about the problem." This is the other side of the coin, and I found it quite heartening. Nevertheless, I think the degree of public acceptance is still considerably wanting.

No Single Answer

Getting back to the proposition that we have many different problems, I think it is altogether unfortunate that some people who have enough experience with social programs to know better have advocated one or another proposal as *the* single answer to our social needs, especially to the problem of lingering poverty.

I would insist that since the reasons for poverty are legion, we need not one, but many approaches if we are to move as rapidly as possible toward its elimination. I hasten to add that I agree with Dr. Burns that while the elimination of poverty is one important objective of social programs, it is not their only legitimate goal. Dr. Burns has said, and I agree, that the success of these programs should not be judged on the basis of benefit/cost analysis or what I would call the "bang for a buck" notion, the bang being the statistical impact of a given program on poverty; social security should aim, as Dr. Burns says, not just at the elimination of poverty through the provision of some minimum income, but also at assurance of the maintenance of some specified fraction of previous incomes.

Dr. Burns says that in the past there has been more emphasis on the second objective; I would maintain that there is growing recognition of the first as well. In the past the emphasis in social insurance has been on the "insurance" aspect; now there is increasing recognition of the "social" side.

I also find myself in agreement with the emphasis which Eveline Burns and Henry Chase have placed on work. Like her, I find little to support the gloomy (or, depending on one's point of view, optimistic) forecasts that automation will in a short space of time make employment an anachronism. On the contrary, there is every indication that for many years to come, probably for decades, and perhaps even for centuries, an overwhelming percentage of people will derive the greatest part of their income from work.

In reference to the point that Henry Chase makes, I think that work will take up a significant though perhaps a slowly declining part of the individual's days, weeks, years, and lifetime. If we are going to have increased leisure, it will perhaps come from earlier retirement, but not by any means exclusively in the form of earlier retirement.

Maximizing Income from Work

If what I have said is true, then we should tie problems of income maintenance and the elimination of poverty as much as possible to those solutions which stress maximizing income from present or past work. In my opinion, the most promising avenues to assuring decent incomes to the largest part of our population are, first, employment at adequate wages and, second, adequate benefit levels under work-related social insurance programs. Moreover, since ours is a work-oriented culture, programs which in one way or another have a work connotation, whether the work relates to the present or to the past, are most likely to win the greatest measure of public support.

I do not agree with everything Henry Chase says, but I think we should take into account to the extent that we can the views he and others express. We should also take into account the views of Congressmen, of the Ways and Means Committee, of the Senate Finance Committee, and so on in trying to achieve the objectives of organized labor and of the liberal community in general. In so doing we stand a better chance of achieving our objectives than if we look for solutions which are completely unacceptable to all these people.

Those solutions to cope with poverty, those solutions for income maintenance which relate in some way to work are those likely to obtain the greatest support. Thus I agree entirely with Dr. Burns's stress on providing enough jobs at rates of pay significantly higher than the poverty minimum and, specifically, with her stress on instituting a program or series of programs assuring such jobs.

I would take issue with her statement that this would be a rounding out of our system of social security, but perhaps this is only a matter of terminology. I would not consider a work program of the kind I think she is talking about and the kind I am talking about as a program of social security. Nevertheless, I agree with her that our objective should be to provide employment at decent wages for the largest number of people, and I am glad to see that she endorses the O'Hara bill approach of providing employment in much-needed public service jobs in the fields of health, education, social welfare, and so on.

In the face of her support for employment in such jobs at wage rates significantly above poverty levels, I cannot understand why she—or so I take it—wishes to eliminate the statutory minimum wage. Rather than eliminate the minimum wage, I would extend its coverage and improve its level. Our objective should be to make sure that each person, whether employed on a private or a public job or in a new public service employment program, receives at least the minimum wage, which should be, as Dr. Burns says, significantly above the poverty level. This should be at least $2.00 an hour at 1969 levels. In other words, there is no reason why we should any longer tolerate the continued existence of the working poor in American society.

Need to Expand and Strengthen Social Insurance

Employment at decent wages must be supplemented by work-related social insurance for the largest possible proportion of those in households whose breadwinner can no longer work, either temporarily or permanently, or is dead. Certainly we have by no means realized the full potential of social security for this purpose. While coverage under Old Age, Survivors, and Disability Insurance and related systems will be close to 100 per cent early in the 1970's, coverage under unemployment insurance and workmen's compensation is much less. In addition, disability insurance under social security should be broadened to include the occupationally disabled. Benefits under all these programs should be raised considerably so that all or nearly all recipients will be above poverty levels.

In this connection I would take issue with the suggestion made by Dr. Burns and others (including Pechman, Aaron, and Taussig in their Brookings Institution study) that the much-needed infusion of government revenues required for adequate financing of our social insurance programs should be earmarked for the minimum benefit. I think there is a danger in the double-decker philosophy which has been espoused by Dr. Burns, the Brookings study, and others.

It seems to me that this is largely a matter of bookkeeping. The fathers of social security predicted the need for the infusion of government revenue into the social security system by about the mid-1960's to take care of what is called the past-service liability. From the viewpoint of winning the maximum public support, what we should be doing is getting over the idea that we need to improve the system in a lot of different ways; that we have to pay for people whose contributions have been much less than the benefits they have received in the past; that the government revenue will be used to finance needed improvements in the entire system. This is the best way of getting public support for the much-needed government contribution from general revenues, whereas singling out the poorest people and saying we are going to take money from other people to pay for them is not.

**Further Supports to Work-Related
Income and Social Insurance**

To return to the central problem posed by Dr. Burns: If the multipronged approach to the whole problem of income maintenance is implemented, most people would be assured of above-poverty incomes through earnings from work or, if there is no longer a breadwinner, from social insurance payments related to previous work. The residual group would then include a relatively few working people who fall through the crevices of social insurance. By far the largest number in this residual group would be nonworking and largely nonemployable mothers and children.

There would also remain the problems faced by some larger-than-average families for whom regular incomes are not sufficient to meet family needs. Family allowances might be one possible way of dealing with the special problem of large families, provided that such allowance payments, first, do not serve as an excuse to depress wages; and, second, are not regarded as a substitute for employment or other welfare or social service programs. Speaking realistically, such allowances are unlikely to be high enough to have a major impact on family incomes.

If I have presented a reasonable analysis of the problem, I do not understand why we must then turn to such a new and little-understood tool as a universal demogrant. Dr. Burns has not indicated exactly where or in what proportion it fits into the whole gamut of income maintenance programs. At any rate, she thinks, as I do, that it is not likely to be achieved very soon. Therefore, what I consider far preferable is for us to try to win public support for the idea that society must accept responsibility for providing decent incomes for nonworking dependents who have no other resources by means of the much-improved public assistance program Dr. Burns advocates and I wholeheartedly support.

Finally, let me endorse Dr. Burns's concluding admonition that we have in our minds the general direction in which we want to move so that we have some criteria against which to measure proposals and programs. This does not mean a single, simple solution which will rid the more fortunate members of society of the problem of the poverty of some less fortunate fellow citizens. Rather we must strive by every means we can command, simple or complex, to make it possible for all people to live in reasonable comfort, security, and dignity—by their own efforts, if possible, but, if not, with the necessary assistance provided in a manner acceptable to those helped and to the rest of the community.

Comment

Michael K. Taussig

I find it very difficult to comment on Dr. Burns's paper. I agree enthusiastically with the body of it, and I disagree on many matters.

Areas of Agreement

I agree very strongly with most of the positions taken by Dr. Burns. I should take this opportunity to express the debt Professor Aaron, Dr. Pechman and I owe her; we found her writing to be original and very helpful in our work on our book.

To record some of the specific points of agreement I have with Dr. Burns: First, I agree with her strongly on the importance of the distinction between the terms "social security" and "social insurance." Unfortunately, in recent years confusion about this difference has been all too prevalent.

I agree very strongly with Dr. Burns that we need government action to provide attractive employment opportunities and more social services as part of a true social security program. I am not sure Dr. Burns considers this to be the really radical step that it is, but it is one of the few radical suggestions with which I thoroughly agree. As far as Bert Seidman's point relating such action to the minimum wage, I suggest that if we had a program which provided jobs for everyone who wanted one, at an attractive wage, a minimum wage would not hurt, but it would be superfluous.

I further agree strongly with Dr. Burns that there should be general revenue financing of all programs intended to alleviate poverty. It seems to me to make no sense whatsoever to tax people who are poor themselves to bring other poor people out of poverty.

I agree with Dr. Burns (this is a somewhat lesser point) that the scope of the state unemployment insurance programs should be limited, and that there should be a clear separation of the dual functions of OASDI. I see both unemployment insurance and OASDI as having two distinct functions (and I am just repeating her points). On the one hand, they involve compulsory budgeting for the middle classes. I am all in favor of that. I think it is a very important objective. I do not downgrade it in any way, but it is a separate objective from the objective of preventing poverty.

Disagreements on Alternatives to Public Assistance

My point of disagreement concerns the type of program that should be used in place of public assistance, how we are to go about bringing people out of poverty and preventing poverty.

It seems to me that Dr. Burns draws too sharp a distinction between what she calls a demogrant or children's allowance and a negative income tax. I should preface my remarks by saying that I am not an uncritical apologist for a negative income tax. I would not advocate without qualification a program that has never been tried. I am involved in a pilot program (initiated in 1968) to test a negative income tax, and I think that should be done. I am not advocating at the present time that we adopt a full-blown negative income tax system—at least not one sufficient to take everybody out of poverty. I do think that a negative income tax program with more modest goals is something very desirable at the present time.

Specifically, Dr. Burns maintains that a universal demogrant is essentially different from a negative income tax. Some of the points she makes involve administrative details that are difficult to evaluate in the absence of concrete specifications. A negative income tax need not necessarily be administered by the Internal Revenue Service; I can see some good reasons why it should not be. In fact, I think the way one should approach these problems is to assume that the same agency (a new agency, perhaps) would administer one or the other program, whichever is selected as the better choice.

I would argue that Dr. Burns's universal demogrant is really a variety of the negative income tax. Essentially, it involves a guaranteed level of income for everyone which a universal negative income tax payment would also provide; and the specific income level guaranteed need not differ. Both involve an implicit or explicit tax on other income. This is unequivocally clear in the case of the negative income tax. But, as I understand it, Dr. Burns's universal demogrant also involves tax rate. It is implicit; perhaps not as easy to see, but there.

Drawbacks of the Demogrant Proposal

The universal demogrant has certain disadvantages. Suppose that the universal demogrant involved a $500 per capita payment, which is probably a very inadequate sum, providing only a $2,000 payment for a family of four—only about half the poverty line in 1970 (if the poverty line had been adjusted as it should have been in the past few years). A $500 payment to everyone (i.e., to each of 200 million persons) would involve a gross cost of $100 billion of additional expense.

Roughly $80 billion of that would go to people above the level of income which makes them liable to personal federal income taxes today, i.e., above the level of minimum deduction plus exemptions depending on family size. That is a rough estimate, but I think it is in the right order of magnitude, good enough for my present purpose.

So this program involves a gross cost of $100 billion additional taxes that have to be collected to finance the demogrant. At the same time, it adds about $80 billion to taxable income. As a public finance student, this suggests to me that the average tax rate required to collect the necessary revenue for the extra $80 billion would probably have to be double or triple the present rate for the personal income tax. If Dr. Burns really believes that this does not affect incentives—she seems to be saying that we should not concern ourselves with incentives when designing an income maintenance program—I suggest she is mistaken. Instead of marginal tax rates ranging from 14 per cent to 70 per cent, I would guess that the financing of her plan would involve marginal tax rates ranging from 30-40 per cent to 140-150 per cent; and I submit that this would affect incentives very greatly.

For the people below the poverty line, the implicit tax rate would be 0 per cent up to the exemption and minimum deduction level, and then would simply become the marginal tax rate under the positive income tax above that level. But it would not be the nice 14 per cent and 15 per cent and 16 per cent that now exists, because in order to finance the program, the government would have to raise all those marginal tax rates; in fact, it would have to raise them up to the level roughly comparable to the levels now contemplated for a negative income tax.

I conclude that the universal demogrant is a negative income tax of a sort that has certain disadvantages in comparison with a straightforward negative income tax.

Dr. Burns suggests a not-so-universal demogrant as a possible substitute, one perhaps limited to the aged, the disabled, and children. This would avoid some of the problems I have just mentioned. The cost would be much less; much less drastic change in the personal income tax would be required to finance it; and so on. I oppose this because I believe that any income maintenance program should be perfectly general and should cover the whole population. I do not believe that it is feasible or moral to specify in advance the "legitimate" causes of poverty. It sounds very convincing to say that the aged, the disabled, and children are special cases which deserve special programs, but there are other people who have other kinds of problems that cannot be specified in advance, and I see no reason to think they are less deserving.

I think the danger involved in specifying particular groups has been well pointed out for us by the history of social insurance and public assistance. We all have come to know OASDI benefits as "earned" benefits and therefore as involving no stigma to the recipients. By way of contrast, public assistance benefits are widely considered as "degrading." I submit this is so only because Congress in 1935 defined these programs in such a way that those to be aided by public assistance were thereby set off from the mass of "normal" Americans. The results, though unforeseen, should teach us not to create a similar situation with respect to children's allowances, whereby people who receive children's allowances are people who "deserve" their benefits, whereas other poor people are "undeserving" and are eligible only for public assistance.

May Dr. Burns, whose position I share in so many respects, meet with only such limited disagreement as is expressed in my comments.

6   Delivery of Health Care: Do We Know Where We Are Going?

Herman M. Somers

It seems to me more useful to open up an array of issues in the delivery of health services than to explore in detail any single aspect, however much such an exploration might happen to interest me. An obvious disadvantage to this approach is that none of the problems I pose can be accompanied by adequate data or analysis, but there is an advantage that may outweigh the handicaps: My approach here should underscore the interlocking dependency of the various elements of health service. It is, I hope, provocative of thought in all quarters, and probably provoking in some—in short, a smorgasbord of ideas.

Prices, Utilization, and Cost

By any available measure, the health services industry has emerged as one of the largest, more rapidly expanding, and most important in the United States. Certainly it is so in terms of total costs, number of persons employed, and amount of government expenditures. Its influence on other economic, social, and political institutions has grown correspondingly. Concomitantly, the character of that growth has become the subject of wide-ranging public policy controversy. Despite that, it remains as a whole, as a system, the least analyzed important industry in the nation and perhaps the least understood. Scholarship in this area has been as fragmented as the industry and the services it renders.

Total expenditures for health and medical care in fiscal year (FY) 1967-68 reached $53.1 billion, or 6.5 per cent of gross national product (GNP). Only three years earlier the figure was $38.9 billion, or 5.9 per cent of GNP. In FY 1950, expenditures were 4.6 per cent of GNP. In less than two decades, health care thus enlarged its share of GNP by over 41 per cent—at the same time that GNP was enjoying spectacular growth. The rate of increase was accelerating with no signs of abatement.

That this phenomenon is by no means entirely explainable by the increased government share of health expenditures is clear from the fact that in the same eighteen-year period, 1950-67, private consumer expenditures for health services shot up 176 per cent. Even after adjustment is made for changes in the value of the dollar (general prices), per capita consumer spending increased 69 per cent.

Expenditures are, of course, a product of prices and utilization rates. Catapulting prices have been by far the more important factor. Between 1950 and 1967, prices contributed 42 per cent more than did added utilization to the increase in personal health care expenditures. The differential is growing larger. In respect to hospital care, prices rose more than five times as fast as use.

Of course, prices have been going up everywhere. But the differential between general price increases and medical price increases has for over twenty years been pronounced, persistent, and progressive. From 1946 to 1967, medical care prices advanced 125 per cent while the index of all prices rose 71 per cent. By far the major influence was hospital prices, which increased 441 per cent, six times as fast as all prices and more than four times as fast as all services in the consumer price index.

Are there signs that this differential may, after all these years, be slowing down? On the contrary, it is accelerating into higher gear. From 1946 to 1960, medical service prices increased at a compounded annual average of 4.6 per cent while all services were increasing at a 3.9 per cent rate, a difference of 21 per cent. Between 1960 and 1965, the differential moved up to an average of 55 per cent faster. In the two years 1966-1968, when medical service prices leaped up to an unprecedented average annual rate of 7.0 per cent, the difference over all services jumped to 71 per cent.

There is considerable finger-wagging at Medicare and Medicaid for this, as it is fashionable to point to the latest particular phenomenon. The infusions of these immense programs undoubtedly contributed substantially to the recent spiraling, but it is equally clear that they were mainly aggravating influences. The forces of inflationary momentum in the health services economy are more basic and long preceded the advent of the new programs. They are also more profound than the recent wave of hospital wage increases, which seems to be the current favorite scapegoat.

Cost measurement and price indices in the health field are far from precision instruments and can be easily faulted, but the magnitude of the rises shown by every available measure are so uniform and great (there are several measures other than the Consumer Price Index and the increases they show are generally even greater) that they cannot be explained away by statistical shortcomings. There can be little doubt as to the validity of these general trends.

For many of you much of this recital is probably familiar in its essential aspects. That may be part of the difficulty now. Medical prices have been belabored for so long among the *cognoscenti* that a prudent speaker, reluctant to inflict boredom on his audience, is likely to avoid it and seek more original subjects. Being tired, and perhaps also despairing, of confrontation with the relentless replication of the data year after year, we are in danger of finally accepting the phenomenon as an unfortunate but inevitable fact of life. If the act goes on long enough it assumes an appearance of having been ordained.

This has a tendency to obscure the vast and ramified consequences of uncontrolled skyrocketing costs in some comfortable but misguided view that "it's only money," and in a declining awareness that the cost trend may be injurious to access, quality, and even health itself—despite easy assumptions that more money automatically leads to improvement. It may be a partial explanation of why, aside from various forms of hand-wringing, very little has been done to contain the burgeoning threat.

Ironically, and not by design, both public and private policy are in the main nurturing the forces of inflation and the disjunctions and waste that are both its cause and effects, in a circular momentum. Our national faith in money as the one certified method of coping with problems has its charms, but is not always valid. I do not advocate parsimony, nor am I a devotee of balanced budgets. The question is where and how we use the money. It may be time to heed the perceptive warning of Harvard economist John T. Dunlop:

> The real function of the cost increases of the past decade, and those in process, should be to compel vast structural changes in the organization of medical care. Nothing could be worse in our society today than to say we need another three to five billion for medical care, and then simply duplicate or multiply the arrangements that we now have. This would get us nowhere. It is the fundamental transformation in a variety of our arrangements that I think is signalled by these cost changes. The permanent problem is the need for more productivity ... brought about by structural changes in the practice and organization of medicine.[1]

In the main we have been duplicating and multiplying the arrangements we already know eat up a large part of each additional dollar by inflation. More than that, we have, through undisciplined support and subsidy, been financially bolstering and perpetuating unsatisfactory arrangements. We have been rapidly stimulating demand on a system, or nonsystem, which is clearly ill-designed to absorb that demand effectively. It then becomes natural to assert scarcity in supply as our difficulty and say we should be spending more to cure that. At the same time our experts point out that we may already be overbuilt with hospital beds in many major communities—and low occupancy rates appear to confirm the contention—and that the nonsystem of health care is so profligate in its use of personnel that, although more manpower is surely needed, even massive increases in numbers of personnel will not avert crises. We had a manpower "crisis" in 1950, when hospitals were employing an average of 1.8 personnel per bed, and the "crisis" is said to be still with us even though in 1969 there were 2.7 personnel per bed, an increase of 50 per cent. There is a high-level bureau in the Public Health Service responsible for medical manpower planning and use, but there is no apparent connection between it and the agencies responsible for the large programs that deliver health services.

Government spent over $14 billion in 1967 for personal health services, 32.5 per cent of all such expenditures. The great bulk came from the federal level, and most of that was in the form of purchase from private providers. The amount and the proportionate impact upon the health care economy is growing fast. Yet, for the most part, the methods of payment have not been accompanied by constraints on prices or substantial attempts to improve the effectiveness of the industry from which the purchasing must be done. (The concept of extended-care facilities and home health services advanced by the Medicare legislation are exceptions to the generalization.) On the contrary, payment methods in our largest programs appear to build in disincentives for price restraint and system effectiveness.

Under Medicare and Medicaid, hospitals are paid their "reasonable costs." In practice, reasonable costs are actual costs, whatever they may turn out to be. Other third parties follow a similar course. Many hospitals now have firm guarantees of reimbursement of 85 per cent or more of their total operating costs. Under the circumstances, management's bargaining posture dissolves against wage and salary demands and staff demands for additional equipment and amenities. There is little, if any, fiscal incentive for management to resist: "It doesn't cost anything." The managerial ineffectiveness of hospitals has been widely publicized. But where are the rewards for greater effectiveness? Daily service rates increased almost 20 per cent in 1967.

In no other realm of economic life are payments guaranteed for costs that are neither controlled by competition nor regulated by public authority, and in which no incentives for economy can be discerned. Yet the criticism is easier to make than is finding an alternative. Is it possible to develop monetary incentives where there is no profit motivation? What might be substituted? Congress has authorized experimentation with incentive reimbursement formulas and the Social Security Administration is planning to go forward with a few. This should be encouraged, even though there is considerable understandable skepticism about the character of proposals which have thus far come in. They are almost inevitably structured on the conventional economic model with which Americans are familiar—one in which there is an identifiable unit product, a profit motivation, or competitive factors. Generally these are not characteristics of our hospital system.

Medicare pays physicians a "reasonable charge" for each service. The guideline is merely that the amount should not exceed the physician's "customary" charge for the particular treatment and that it be within the range of fees "prevailing" in the community for similarly situated doctors. There is little to prevent a doctor from raising his customary fees. And, of course, increases in customary fees will automatically raise the prevailing levels. Prevailing fees more than doubled their previous long-term rate of increase in both 1966 and 1967. Now we are also witnessing the crumbling of the few and modest restraints that had existed in Blue Shield reimbursement plans. They are announcing plans for adoption of "customary" and "usual fee" standards.

Nonetheless, as everybody knows, the hospitals are complaining vigorously that they are being shortchanged, that present reimbursements do not fully meet costs. The main contention is that the formula provides only for current operating costs and not for capital needs. They are actively gunning—and they are skilled gunners in this field—for augmentation of all third-party reimbursements to pay for capital as well. Another suggested device is for government to supply long-term loans for construction and renovation. Since reimbursement would then be expected to include allowances for interest and amortization, essentially this would have the same outcome as the first proposal.

Another possibility is direct government grants, on the lines of a massively expanded Hill-Harris program, thus detaching these capital costs from reimbursement claims. This has the advantage of at least permitting more effective selectivity in allocation of capital and not allowing each hospital to be the sole judge of its own capital needs, which then become in effect a tax upon the entire community. Despite the wide publicity given to "planning," this is still the prevailing practice. All these proposals have the disadvantage of reducing the traditional dependence of hospitals upon raising funds through community participation, giving the population to be served an opportunity to give or withhold approval of hospital policy.

It is not denied that there is a genuine problem of capital, particularly for renovation of obsolete and run-down facilities. But, under present conditions, in all proposed methods of further government and third-party payments, cost restraints are even further diminished.

I close this section by alluding breifly to a probelm which is, or ought to be, just over the horizon, to which virtually no systematic attention has been directed. It has already been indicated that the proportion of the nation's resources expended for health care is rising spectacularly. How far can it or should it go? The Report of the National Advisory Commission on Health Manpower blithely tells us that "some experts have predicted an increase from the present 6 to 25 per cent of GNP for health service."[2] The time is not specified and, perhaps to avoid libel, the experts are not identified. Nor is it indicated what portion of the increase will represent actual increases of service and what portion medical price inflation.

It seems highly improbable that the nation will find it acceptable to deny itself so large a proportion of other goods and services, many equally relevant to a good life. It will, of course, be remembered that absolute dollar expenditures can increase considerably even while the proportion of GNP stands still. So we are not talking about a freeze on dollars but about the nature of allocation of the nation's total resources. The Commission on Health Manpower figure correctly indicates that technological advances in medicine and other factors will make the health industry able to consume whatever amount of money we are willing to pour into it. But is there a more objective way of determining how much is optimal?

Even if we shut our eyes to other legitimate human goals and confine ourselves to maximizing health objectives, we must keep in view that the health level of a family or a community is not merely the product of the quality and quantity of direct health services used. Health is also significantly related to levels of income and education, recreation, housing, air and water supply, food, and so on. With improvement of health as the objective, as we reach higher levels of health investment it becomes increasingly unclear whether a given economic input into health facilities or services will move us more or less readily toward that goal than a similar input in education, housing, or recreation. Can we develop the technical skills to cope with that formidable problem?

A similar question arises in respect even to direct health care investment. We have seen that annual expenditures already exceed $53 billion and are going up. Needless to say, the private sector of this vast outlay is unplanned and unprogrammed. Even the government portion, about 37 per cent and rising, has not been appraised as a whole but is an array of independently determined fragments. The relative effectiveness of different distributions of the health dollar over the range of health activities—construction, research, hospital care, physicians, public health activities, education,* and so forth—has never been analyzed. In the light of limited resources, does this too not demand some cost-effectiveness analysis? Are we developing the criteria and the tools?

*The costs of medical education are omitted from all health and medical cost data used in this presentation.

Quality

How much health is all our additional investment buying? How effective are the services? The question of quality is as crucial as it is elusive. Unfortunately, we have not yet learned how to measure the output. Such indices as we have relate primarily to input—the character of institutions, training of personnel, types of procedures employed, and the like. As this is the best we have, we should at least make the most of that. We do not.

It is only recently that many of our states have adopted hospital licensing laws, and many of these only under pressure of eligibility requirements for Hill-Burton funds. Many of the licensing laws are virtually free of quality standards and are related only to the ordinary safety and health hazards of the structure. Purely voluntary action, by professional societies, created the accreditation program of the Joint Commission on Accreditation of Hospitals (JCAH). Many hospitals failed to meet even these admittedly minimal standards and there were few apparent consequences for not receiving accreditation.

Perhaps the single greatest advance in hospital standards was brought about by the Medicare legislation. It provided that fulfilling at least JCAH standards would be a condition of participation. For the first time, on a national basis, significant economic leverage accompanied standard-setting. Hundreds of hospitals were obliged to upgrade themselves substantially. Unfortunately, the law requires that Medicare accept the fact of JCAH accreditation as conclusive evidence that the standards are in fact being met. There is evidence that this is not always the case. The capacities of JCAH for protecting its own standards are severely limited. It employs less than twenty full-time physicians to cover some 4,000 accredited institutions. Normally surveys are made every three years and these are acknowledged to be less than thorough. State agencies report that not infrequently JCAH-accredited hospitals do not actually fully meet Medicare standards, which are certainly moderate. Fortunately, the JCAH leadership is aware of the shortcoming and promises steps to strengthen effectiveness. Whether it will be able to muster the resources to do so remains to be seen.

Medicare is also authorized to set standards for independent laboratories, suppliers of portable X-ray services, and out-patient physical therapy services. Quality levels have been improved in all these areas, profiting the entire population and not only Medicare beneficiaries. This has not been accomplished without a struggle. Resistance, particularly among nursing homes, continues to be active.

But in the critical field of physician services, Medicare has no authority to establish standards. Any licensed physician is fully eligible to participate in the program. Very few would, I believe, try to defend state licensing procedures as adequate. Among other difficulties, a license once granted is good for life, whether the doctor does or does not engage in actual practice. In an age of specialization demanded by advanced technology, any licensed doctor can undertake any kind of procedure in the entire medical field. The only substantial protection we have against these dangerous potentials is the staff regulations of good hospitals. But these regulations do not control what happens outside the hospital and, of course, thousands of doctors have no hospital affiliation at all and carry on a full practice nevertheless.

The irony of this aspect of the Medicare law is illustrated by an actual recent event. A hospital was disqualified from participation in the program on dramatic evidence of improper and hazardous procedures and practices. The program would no longer pay the hospital for any services it rendered, but at the same time it is obliged to pay the individual physicians who own and operate the hospital for any individual medical services they may render Medicare patients in or out of hospital. They have licenses.

But Medicare cannot be held up as the bad example. Other third-party payors have no standards either. There are at least clear signs that the Social Security Administration is seriously troubled by the anomalous situation and plans to take steps toward coping with the problem. The agency plans to seek legislation that would enable the program to discontinue reimbursement for services of a physician when there is evidence of fraud, repeated overcharging, or a pattern of rendered services substantially in excess of those justified by sound medical practice. It is also studying means of excluding from program reimbursement the services of a practitioner who has repeatedly rendered and billed for services or supplies which are harmful to the patient or grossly inferior by professional standards. The agency does not have the authority to exclude a physician from the program on any of these grounds.

There are many signs that the plethora of money pouring into health institutions is not always conducive to elevating quality. Hospitals are known to expand prestige services which they are incapable of performing adequately. Martin Cherkasky has pointed out that New York has twice as many centers of cardiac surgery as it needs, with the result that the costs are "astronomical" and the quality "miserable."[3] The President's Commission on Heart Disease, Cancer, and Stroke confirmed that this is not a purely local phenomenon. It reported that 30 per cent of the 777 hospitals equipped to do closed-heart surgery had no such cases in the year under study. Of all hospitals equipped to do open-heart surgery, 41 per cent averaged under one per month. Little of this work was of an emergency nature and the mortality rate for both procedures was "far higher . . . than in institutions with a full work load."[4]

As I have said, we do not have any adequate measure of the changes in quality resulting from all our expenditures, but the superficial signs offer a basis for more concern than has been evidenced. Economist Victor R. Fuchs, in his keynote address at the 1967 National Conference on Medical Costs, said:

Although we spend much more per person for medical care than any other country, the blunt truth is that we do not enjoy the highest health levels. On the contrary, many European countries have age-specific death rates considerably below our own. The relatively high infant mortality rate in this country is disturbing, and difficult to explain. The disparity in death rates for middle-aged males is even more shocking, and has more serious economic implications. In the United States, of every 100 males who reach the age of 45, only 90 will reach 55; in Sweden the comparable rate is 95. During this critical decade when most men are at the peak of their earning power, the U. S. death rate is double the Swedish rate, and higher than that of almost every Western nation. It certainly seems legitimate to ask why.[5]

The relatively low health status cited by Fuchs does not mean that the finest medical care is not available in the United States or that our doctors or hospitals are inferior. Nor does it mean that we spend less proportionately for health than other nations; the contrary is true. It does mean that our well-advertised magnificent resources are distributed very inequitably, that the country has both excellent and very poor quality of care. The head of the Health Affairs Office of the Office of Economic Opportunity has noted: "At this moment, the United States stands 15th among the nations of the world in infant mortality rates. It is our 30 million poor who primarily account for our unfavorable position."

It would be a mistake, however, to assume that the problem lies exclusively in the inability of the poor to purchase care. The evidence is ample that even when given the means of purchase they get bad care. And this experience is not confined to the poor by any means.

Despite frequent pronouncements that health care is a civic right to which all people are entitled regardless of economic position, and despite the amplification of government programs for low-income families, the fact remains that by every measure the poor are severely disadvantaged in the quality and quantity of care they receive. Whatever the merits of the maxim "The sick get poorer and the poor get sicker," there is an indisputable statistical association of increased morbidity and mortality with poverty.

Government has been increasing its programs and expenditures for the poor. If money alone were the answer, there should be a very significant impact. It is estimated that in fiscal 1968 public expenditures for health services for the poor exceeded $11 billion, most of it for the aged. It should not, however, be assumed that the poor can be provided with the medical care they need if only government stands ready to pay their bills; Medicaid is the most recent of the unintended case studies to make that point. There is a formidable array of barriers to care confronting the poor, including, in addition to inability to pay, such factors as the paucity of good facilities and qualified professionals in ghettos and rural areas, racial discrimination in provision of services, attitudes of health personnel and institutions toward "charity" cases, and the inhibited, fearful, and uninformed attitudes of the poor themselves toward medical care. Most important, however, is the fragmented system of delivery of services which prevails for most of the health economy, but which negatively affects the poor in particular.

Delivery of Services and Planning

Sparked by the cost pressures, an extraordinary, and often bewildering, assortment of investigations and reports of official and expert bodies have been made. No matter what the composition of the particular body or the point of departure for the inquiry, all the results underline Professor Dunlop's thesis quoted above. The virtually uniform view expressed is that underlying each particular problem is the disorganization and fragmentation of health services, the general lack of system.

For example, the National Advisory Commission on Health Manpower found that the inadequacies in health manpower could not be successfully tackled outside of reform of the institutional framework within which the manpower is employed. It reported:

> There *is* a crisis in American health care. . . . *The crisis, however, is not simply one of numbers.* It is true that substantially increased numbers of health manpower will be needed over time. But if additional personnel are employed in the present manner and within the present patterns and "systems" of care, they will not avert or even perhaps alleviate the crisis. *Unless we improve the system* through which health care is provided, care will continue to become less satisfactory, even though there are massive increases in costs and numbers of personnel. . . .
>
> Medicine has participated in the general explosion of science and technology, and possesses cures and preventives that could not have been predicted even a decade ago. But the organization of health services has not kept pace with advances in medical science or with changes in society itself. Medical care in the United States is more a collection of bits and pieces (with overlapping, duplication, great gaps, high costs, and wasted effort), than an integrated system in which needs and efforts are closely related.[6]

In a similar vein, commenting on President Johnson's warning that by the mid-1970's the United States would need twice as many health care personnel as it required in 1968, the knowledgeable President of the Blue Cross Association of America, Walter J. McNerney, said, "We would get more bang for the buck if we put relatively more emphasis on organization, financing, and design of the health system than simply producing professional manpower."[7]

The report of the able Barr Committee (the Department of Health, Education, and Welfare Secretary's Advisory Committee on Hospital Effectiveness) also placed heavy emphasis on this point; it stated that "the key fact about the health service as it exists today is . . . disorganization," accompanying the assertion with concrete proposals for countervailing action.[8] The National Advisory Commission on Health Facilities also stressed the need for system. To my knowledge, there was no follow-up on any of these reports after they were delivered. One may be led to wonder why they were commissioned. It's that kind of field.

There is a remarkable degree of agreement on necessary general objectives, and much less, of course, on specific details. There is even less agreement on how substantial reform can be achieved in view of the scattered authority and influence in the field. The central focus is upon the need to apply modern technology to the delivery of care and the need to systematize its far-flung component parts. This view is most often expressed in the terms "comprehensive health care system" and "planning." There are considerable differences in regard to what the terms mean or ought to mean. Unfortunately they have taken on some of the attributes of convenient slogans rather than programmatic guidelines.

We have seen considerable stir in government regarding this issue—a veritable bedlam of conferences, meetings, reports, and talk. A new agency has been born, the National Center for Health Services Research and Development. It is too young for any judgment to be made. Among the action programs in this area, the most prominent are the regional medical programs (RMP), and the comprehensive health planning legislation often referred to as the 749 program (Public Law 89-749). Both have thus far proved disappointing to those who envisaged them as moving toward a reordering and systematizing of health services. As is often true in legislation and administration, the machinery devised has not proved consonant with the objectives.

RMP was intended to help bridge the gap between scientific advance and delivery of its product in medical services by encouraging regional coordination between large medical centers and research institutions, on the one hand, and community hospitals and the myriad small health units and individual practitioners on the other. The nation is now covered by RMP organizations. With rare exceptions, their projects are not directed toward regionalization or restructuring systems of delivery. Some interesting and useful things are being done in various fields, such as the continuing education of physicians, the training and upgrading of nurses and specialized personnel, and the investigation of methods of treatment for cardiac patients. But, for the most part, the central objective has been lost sight of or despaired of. Discussion of the operational reasons for that development must be left for some other occasion.

Almost everybody in the health field now gives verbal endorsement to planning in some form. Government has promoted the principle for a long time. The Blue Cross Association has supported it. The American Hospital Association has recently given official endorsement, although with a hard bargaining, quid pro quo condition. The American Medical Association has stated support for local voluntary planning bodies. There is no agreed-upon definition of objectives, but ideally and oversimply, the purposes of planning might be said to be to achieve a more rational organization of health services in the community and nation in the interest of greater effectiveness, i.e., greater accessibility and improved quality at reasonable cost. Many supporters would declare more modest objectives.

The Hill-Burton Hospital Survey and Construction Act of 1946 was the nation's first significant instrumentality for a limited form of planning. An attempt was made to relate federal grants to state-wide plans, based upon an inventory of existing facilities and needs. Starting in 1960, the U. S. Public Health Service began to render financial support to local and state planning bodies. About seventy or more such bodies have come into being, covering geographic areas that probably encompass more than half the population of the country. Mainly they are concerned with new construction or expansion of institutional facilities, primarily hospitals. They are generally voluntary nongovernmental bodies with no formal authority, with the result that in most instances the enterprises must be judged as valuable educational experience on the way to effective action. Only New York and Rhode Island have moved to a program of legally enforceable planning.

Apparently one of the objectives of the comprehensive health planning legislation was to universalize the movement and to enlarge its horizons. Its authors sought to conteract the conspicuous shortcoming of the existing planning bodies by introducing some new concepts, including more emphasis on consumer and community participation in planning bodies, more emphasis on ambulatory care, broadening coverage to include a variety of health-related fields, and more emphasis on public accountability.

Unfortunately, to judge by the outcome thus far, the law seems to have thrown out the baby with the bathwater. It has seriously disabled and demoralized the pre-existing and evolving health facilities planning bodies, which naturally have assumed that Public Law 89-749 was the signal for their gradual termination, and no practical program has replaced them. It structured the new state bodies in a manner to diminish the only practical power base for health planning, the hospitals or medical centers which had nurtured the old bodies, and left a power vacuum. The new legislation did nothing to encourage the correction of the greatest shortcoming of the existing bodies, as pointed out by the Barr Committee and others—the lack of any enforcement powers.

The states have established their 749 planning organizations, under the requirement of the federal legislation, but they understandably still have no clear notion of what it was the federal authorities expected them to do. I say "understandably" from personal experience as a member of one state health planning council who has often raised the question and found that Washington ain't telling. Thus far most of the stated bodies are in a limbo quite detached from any meaningful involvement in actual health delivery activities in their states. As Anne Somers put it recently,

> What influence have these bodies had on the actual financing and organization of care in their jurisdictions? Have they helped to shape or improve the states' Medicaid programs? Or their mental health programs? Or their workmen's compensation programs? Have they concerned themselves with health insurance standards and rates in their states? Or with the distribution of physician services in any meaningful way? Have they even tried?
>
> At the local level there is even less to show. A number of the area-wide planning bodies do have some influence in hospital programs and developments. But in the mish-mash of so-called planning activity going on today in some of our large cities with OEO, 749, 239, Model Cities, and area-wide planning bodies competing with each other for limited staff and funds and for the time and attention of hospital administrators and physicians, it is no wonder that the very concept of planning is becoming discredited. To the "non-system" of health care . . . has been added a layer of "non-planning." Confusion has been confounded.[9]

Are things better in Washington? What influence does the Office of Comprehensive Health Planning, despite its grand title, have on the operations of Medicare, or the Federal Employees Health Benefits Program, or the Veterans Administration programs? These federal programs are vital segments of the health care economy. But there is no relationship between what goes on in the Office of Comprehensive Planning and what these federal programs do or do not do.

It can, of course, be answered that P. L. 749 was never intended as an instrument of planning at the federal level. That in itself bespeaks a great deal about the realism of the law. The federal government, with its numerous and expanding health programs, must have a planning capability of its own if it is to be persuasive and credible to the states and the private sector it is presumably trying to influence. It has the responsibility for establishing some broad national guidelines and priorities to assist the entire national planning effort.

It seems clear that, at this point in our experience at least, any appraisal of the collectivity of programs presumably intended to help rationalize the structure of medical services and the delivery system—the problems at the heart of our difficulties in health care—must be, regrettably, negative and pessimistic.

Conclusion

If any theme emerges from these wide-ranging observations, it may be this: Twenty years ago, when we were debating President Truman's national health insurance proposals, it was appropriate that our primary concern be with opening the blocked gates of access to health services by removing the financial barriers. With increased affluence, the phenomenal growth of private health insurance, and the vast expansion of government's role, access is no longer the major problem. There are still significant pockets of nonaccess due to finances and these must not and will not be overlooked.

Today, however, we find ourselves with other priority issues which threaten the progress we have achieved in access. Price inflation, if it continues on its present merry flight, could again narrow or close the access gates to those who pay directly for medical care and those who depend on private health insurance. Price inflation threatens the survival of private health insurance.

We cannot successfully cope with either prices or access inadequacies without grappling with the chaotic delivery structure that underlies them. Progress has been made, in that there is now a widespread awareness of and concern with the problem. Never before has health care been so much in the public eye as a personal, community, and public policy problem. But to date we have not proved sufficiently knowledgeable or inventive to develop effective machinery for change. That is our pre-eminent need.

It is commonplace to read in health care literature the familiar warning to different components of the industry that if they do not start to fly right the government may take over. It may be interesting to ask hypothetically just what the government will do if it should take over. Does it know? Do we know what we would want it to do? Perhaps if we did we could find a more effective means for our goals than a take-over.

I find that my remarks have on the whole accented the negative. Many of the observations are intended to offer a controversial basis for discussion, out of which I hope there may arise more affirmation. In any case, I should not want to imply that we should accept discouragement, for that is not my mood. I regard the problems I have recited as an exhilarating challenge for all of us. I am confident that, as a nation, we have the brains, the energy, and the goodwill to meet it.

Notes

1. John T. Dunlop, "The Capacity of the United States to Provide and Finance Expanding Health Service," New York Academy of Medicine *Bulletin,* vol. 41, no. 12 (December 1965), 1326-27.

2. *Report of the National Advisory Commission on Health Manpower* (Washington, D. C.: U. S. Government Printing Office, 1967), vol. II, p. 182.

3. Martin Cherkasky, "Resources Needed to Meet Effectively Expected Demands for Service," New York Academy of Medicine *Bulletin,* vol. 42, no. 12 (December 1966), 1091.

4. *National Program to Conquer Heart Disease, Cancer, and Stroke,* Report to the President (Washington, D. C.: U. S. Government Printing Office, February 1965), vol. II, p. 55.

5. Victor R. Fuchs, "The Basic Forces Influencing Costs of Medical Care," *Report of the National Conference on Medical Costs* (Washington, D. C.: U. S. Department of Health, Education and Welfare, 1968), pp. 16-31.

6. *Report of the National Advisory Commission on Health Manpower,* vol. I, pp. 2-3.

7. Walter J. McNerney, "The Organization and Financing of Health Services," University of Minnesota Lecture Series on Health of the Nation (Minneapolis, July 19, 1968).

8. *Report,* U. S. Department of Health, Education and Welfare (Washington, D. C.: U. S. Government Printing Office, 1968), p. 9.

9. Anne Somers, "Goals into Reality, the Challenges of Health Planning," *Hospitals,* vol. 43 (August 1, 1969), 47.

Comment

Howard Ennes

Let me begin by extending to Professor Rohrlich and his colleagues compliments on focusing on this concept of social economics. I am not quite sure that my perceptions are the same as theirs. But new insights and new perspectives in this area are only too welcome to help us break out of the straitjacket that it seems to me the health Establishment got itself into, and help us to know just where we are right now.

The Field of Health Care: A Closed Society

It seems to me that in essence we have had a closed society in the health area. It has been the province of the professionals. There has been a lot of talk about the needs of the patient and the needs of the people; yet most of the time we seem to think in terms of professional interest and not in terms of the patient's interest or the people's interest. The perspective has been largely that of the convenience of the professional—the disease he wants to study, the condition he wants to treat. It has been a curative instead of a preventative view. It has been in terms of the welfare of the profession. I think all this has probably been with the honest conviction that what they were doing was also best for the patient, but they hardly ever asked the patient whether it was.

We have put the onus for controlling costs on the individual, through deductibles and co-insurance. We speak of over-utilization, and we penalize the patient for what the professional does: The professional, the physician, controls whether or not the patient is in the hospital and how long he stays there. But we penalize the patient for something he does not control. In light of today's hospital charges, that is indeed a $100-a-day misunderstanding.

It seems to me that the whole process is becoming futile—almost immoral—without reasonable facilitation and cooperation by the professionals. It seems to me that controls are needed, backed up by rational, planned systems.

We have been living and are living in a closed society, as far as health care is concerned; we need merely look at what has happened, for example, in the field of health insurance to see this. In the formative years of health insurance, perhaps thirty years ago, we in the health insurance business were very diffident. We thought we knew our business insofar as it concerned risk-taking, money transfer, claims administration, and fiscal management; but we did not think we knew very much about the medical field and so we deferred to the professionals.

Now we are beginning to realize that we were looking at the problem from the wrong angle. We had accepted a sort of noneconomic, pseudomarket concept of health care. We thought that by underwriting workshops for the profession we were making a contribution to health care. Until quite recently, I think, we did not take fully into account the health care needs of the people and we did not feel it was our responsibility to do so. Today perhaps we ought to be thinking about taking on an ombudsman advocacy for the consumer.

This in many ways accounts for our emphasis, until now, on in-patient care—hospitalization, i.e., a system that puts a premium on spending money to keep somebody in a convenient point for the use, literally, of the professional. Of course, this is not health insurance at all, even though we call it that. At best it is hospital insurance, or perhaps sickness insurance.

I do not want to be crude about this, but I do think health is much too important to be left to the professionals alone. I think it is probably also too important to be left to the consumers alone, or to any other category, including the economists. I believe in a partnership approach to understanding needs and resources. Perhaps this new concern with social economics can help us get some hold on the problems of needs, resources and social commitments—get them into some balance, some rational relationship. As Professor Somers has said, health is not the sole product of personal and medical care services. Nor is it merely an end in itself. It is also a means of helping individuals and families achieve a sense of fuller living. Perhaps in our pursuit of social economics, at least as applied to the health field, we might consider values and ends as well as means and costs.

A Somber Picture, With Grounds for Optimism

Professor Somers did not leave many bases uncovered. Like him, I am somewhat ambivalent. I am less sure about my own mood, except that I feel frustrated and impatient. Unsure of what we ought to be doing, I harbor a sense of impending doom. As a matter of fact, I think the insurance industry as a whole is very much concerned about the medical inflation and about the fact that we have not come to grips with this problem at all.

The health care situation is, on the whole, a somber one, even though some of its many dimensions are bright. I am not quarreling with the fact that America does have some of the best *medical* care in the world. But we do not have very good health care for the usual problems that most of us have to deal with on a day-to-day basis, or for those particularly that the less privileged have to deal with. The over-all picture is not a cohesive or integrated composition; it seems to me rather more like a set of overlapping and out-of-focus images reflecting patchwork and piecework efforts to deal (mostly after the fact) with the impact of disease and disability, not with health. The background of the picture is marked by very rapid change—technological, social, emotional—and, obviously, by rising expectations, by runaway costs, and, very importantly, by a growing and ever more apprehensive concern and interest on the part of the consumers.

Despite this somber setting, I would suggest that we can be optimistic, that we can make some progress. I think there are four possible lines of action.

One, which seems obvious to me, is the creation of better living conditions and community services.

The second is a more effective and better organized delivery of health services.

The third is a higher quality of performance by health workers and through the development of new types of health manpower.

The fourth is a more relevant system of health communication and services which will foster improved personal and family health practices.

On these points I touch briefly, critically, and I hope not too cynically.

Health and Ecology

There is really no need to elaborate on the importance of living conditions. Gerard Peil reminds us of a fact we would like to forget, that the real progress we have made in this country, in mortality in particular, has been made because of environmental efforts, and has had very little to do with medical care. There is a great deal more we can do, especially in places like north Philadelphia and south Chicago, in this respect. The documentation is available. The larger issues are issues of human ecology, such as are dealt with by Rene Jules DuBos and in the symposium sponsored by the Consumer Protection and Environmental Health Service.[1]

Another document that points to some of the problem areas is *Social Forces and the Nation's Health—A Task Force Report*. It contains the following passage:

> Protection of the nation's health cannot be secured by the fragmented efforts of separate agencies or communities or by the efforts of a few segments of the population planning and working alone. The health professions alone cannot provide these conditions which are the prerequisites for health:
>   1. The immediate physical living and working conditions, such as housing and transportation systems, which minimize health and safety hazards and facilitate the adoption of sound health habits and practices.
>   2. A larger physical environment, which contributes to rather than threatens people's health by assuring clean air, safe and adequate water supply, reasonable noise level, etc.
>   3. Economic conditions which put such necessities as adequate nutrition, housing and leisure time within everyone's reach.

4. Legal and social systems which allow all citizens full access to resources and opportunities needed if these citizens are to function as healthy, productive members of society.

5. A system for providing high quality health services, facilities, and other resources on the basis of need equally available to all.

6. People who learn and adhere to sound personal health habits and practices in their daily lives so as to assure a normal development and to optimize maintenance of mental and physical health.

7. People who are able and willing to seek and utilize available health services when needed and to follow medical advice and regimen.[2]

On the question of health care delivery system, Professor Somers and I may disagree somewhat—not really on need, but on performance, on implementation. There can be no doubt, it seems to me, that the objective is to provide service where needed, when needed, and under circumstances that are acceptable and appropriate. Nor do I see how one can talk about a delivery system without talking about planning, organization, interrelationships, and rational accountability.

I do think, however, that the national leadership has been a lot smarter than it is commonly believed to have been. It may not have been very adept in communicating. There is irony in the fact that we have been talking for years about the importance of local action, and here is a situation which is literally forcing confrontation of issues at the point where it counts. To be sure, more needs to be done, especially in the setting of clearer goals.

I think it was a mistake not to include in Public Law 89-749 a directive to develop continuing mechanisms for setting national goals. It is my personal conviction that the concept of integrated comprehensive planning cannot be limited to health, but must relate to other aspects that are important. In commenting on those interested in planning, Professor Somers neglects to mention that the private health insurance industry took up the problem of comprehensive planning. It did this in the face of all the pressures from organized medicine and the hospitals and despite the presumed affinity between the providers and financers of the delivery system. Well before Congress passed the comprehensive health planning legislation, we were out working in this area. Our industry now has a fifty-state system of contact and alert points, with the participation of about thirty-five state planning councils.

The important point relative to Public Law 89-749 is that by getting the industry to plug into the process that was beginning to be developed we began to get some input into our program planning and into our policy-making; information that was not there before began flowing into our system. We began to break through the closed system, the closed society that the professionals had built up. We began to get a flow of some new ideas, some new concepts and facts.

I am sure this has initiated a process of change. The fact that private health insurers are now involved in group practice and are actively supporting the planning agencies with manpower and resources has come about as the result of our breakout from the closed society. This change in perception is, I think, crucial, and it is focusing our attention on some of the organizational challenges we are talking about.

Organization and Delivery of Services

The need for organizational change can be epitomized, I think, in terms of one word: quality. We must look at the issue of quality in new dimensions and from new perspectives.

I think we are beginning to witness a process of consumer examination of what is going on, what is being delivered in health care. Specifically, the consumer seems to be concerned about four aspects of care, by which he appears to test the quality of our health services today.

The consumer's first question is: Are the services accessible? This means accessible in time and place and at reasonable cost to individuals, to families, to communities, and to the national economy.

The consumer's second question is: Are the services available (or at least planned for) without serious gaps (one such gap, surely, makes the maternal and infant situation in this country) and (somewhat less important) without too much overlap?

The consumer's third question is whether the facilities, services, and programs are appropriate to individual and family needs, as well as to over-all community needs.

Finally, the consumer asks whether the services are acceptable. I think this is being judged not only in terms that providers of care would apply, notably professional quality, proper organization, and financing, but also by criteria of need the consumers perceive for themselves, including in particular what they deem their inherent right to human dignity. In this regard we have made some horrendous mistakes, albeit with the best of intentions.

Quality of Performance

In the light of these tests, it seems to me we must think in terms of higher quality of performance as the gauge of relevancy. Here is an area which has been influenced substantially by market conditions. Might it be possible, by proper organization of the system, to utilize as incentives in the market those same concerns for involvement, for income, for reason, for satisfaction, for identity that motivate professionals just as they do young people?

In addition, we must be thinking in terms of new, better, and different types of services and of manpower. Let me illustrate. In the experience with neighborhood health centers across the country we find that we can use effectively people from the community as links, to bring people in, interpret to them what the doctor says. These interpreters seem to be capable of furnishing the ingredient that is missing in the whole process of health services delivery: a sense of empathy. As we are finding out in the neighborhood health centers, and as Professor Somers says, without that kind of interest and concern to provide links and bridges with the people who need the services, all the money in the world may not suffice to eliminate bad service or provide effective service.

We need thousands, hundreds of thousands of people for these kinds of jobs. Ideally, the ratio might have to be 1:850—one interpreter, or link, for each bloc of 850 people served. Even at a much higher ratio, auxiliary personnel would still be needed in substantial numbers. What are the implications? Jobs are one: meaningful, important jobs at a cost, on balance, not very much above present welfare expenditures—jobs that offer satisfaction and potential growth. This approach would also contribute to finding a solution to a basic problem of the economy—jobs for untrained people who are nevertheless "professionals," in the business of relating to people, something middle-class professionals seem to have a hard time doing. And perhaps we would also be saving money in the long run if we were to act along these lines on a far larger scale than we have up till now.

Health Communications

My final point pertains to the role of the consumer—or, better, of the individual, the citizen.

I do not think the current concern for participatory democracy is just a fad; the concept strikes me as a redundancy rather than a new notion. If democracy is not involvement and participation, then what are we talking about? But have we put it into practice? In the health field, we have really been only *talking* about involvement and participation, because when the chips were down we *used* people to achieve what we, of course, considered to be "good" ends. The time has come to open the way out of this essentially closed society, to break through in a large way. I think we should begin an open communications process.

P. L. 89-749 seems to assume that somehow consumers would suddenly become experts at communicating and planning, and at relating to one another. Is it not time to seriously consider ways of facilitating this by a concerted nation-wide effort at what for lack of a better term I call community health citizenship? I would expect this to comprise professional preparation, continuing education and related research and development. I think the first priority must be the individual in his sundry capacities: as a member of his community and his family; as a citizen who is an earner and manager, parent, professional, legislator—in other words, each one of us. I think we should also end with the individual and that our purpose should be to facilitate his understanding of his world, of his resources, his opportunities, and his responsibilities.

Probably it would be well to start off with responsibility, which is the other side of the coin of rights. And the right to access to health care is now a political fact of life. (We need to remind ourselves that the demands for rights and the pressure for consumer participation stem from the very unhappy experiences of millions of individuals trying to satisfy their pressing needs.)

First, I think each of us has a responsibility to know himself as a being and to know his environment, social and physical, so that he can be in a position to shape his life style in a way that maximizes his personal options for living fully.

Secondly, there is the responsibility to utilize health services and environmental supports, both personal health services and community health services (I would emphasize environmental elements), and to utilize these with optimal efficiency and economy. Incidentally, getting more people involved in the realities of services might prove more effective than past attempts at systematizing, identifying, and controlling costs.

The third responsibility, one I consider crucial, is to participate constructively in community health and environmental planning, and in the priority-setting and decision-making that goes along with that. If the citizen-consumer is to learn to function constructively along these lines he will need much help.

I do not think we can talk about individual responsibility when either resources or authority are unavailable. Consider, for example, the responsibility of the individual to know himself, particularly the individual in the city, where our problems are most acute. I think Ralph Ellison has put it rather neatly:

> I think one of the things we can do about the city is to look at it, to try to see it not merely as an instrumentality for making money but a place for allowing the individual to achieve his highest promise. With that in mind you would try to construct a city or reconstruct a city in ways which would encourage a more gracious sense of human possibility. You would teach, if at all possible, the immigrants—whether they are black or white or brown—that there is certain knowledge which one must have in order to live in the city without adding too much discomfort to his neighbors.[3]

Although we have barely started to try to do that, I think we could probably be more optimistic than Ellison suggests. Merely avoiding problems is not enough; our concern should be how to facilitate the individual's capacity to cope with and to shape the human condition.

As President Jacqueline Grennan of Hunter College said: "The great need in education is to enable an individual to find his own voice, to speak with it, to stand by it. Learning is not essentially expository, but essentially exploratory."[4] To provide the conditions and the opportunities for the creation of a sense of ecological understanding and exploration is what I mean by the ideal community health citizenship.

In sum, then, in sharp contrast with the character of the present health service picture—the nonsystem of corrective medical care—the new picture of health might have as its central goal a responsibility concerned citizenry prepared to participate effectively in the development and maintenance of a conprehensive system which maximizes the inherent capabilities of each human being for fuller living. I am reasonably optimistic, frankly, despite the gloomy facts. Circumstances are propitious for change, for action. What bothers us all is direction. Which way should be be going? We cannot seem to get many workable answers from just those people who should be supplying them. To engage intelligently in what we call action planning, we must answer the question of relevancy, and do better in establishing goals and identifying needs, than we have. The insurance industry—not only the health insurance industry, but the total insurance industry—is ready to help with money and manpower and implementation. But I do think that the first responsibility is with the professionals, with the people who have taken it upon themselves voluntarily to accept the responsibility of leadership in this field.

Notes

1. *Symposium on Human Ecology,* Airlie House, Warrenton, Va.; November 24-27, 1968 (U.S. Department of Health, Education, and Welfare, Public Health Service, Consumer Protection and Environmental Health Service.

2. *Social Forces and the Nation's Health—A Task Force Report* (U.S. Department of Health, Education, and Welfare, Health Services and Mental Health Administration, May, 1968), pp. 3-4.

3. Ralph Ellison, "The Crisis of Optimism," in *The City of Crisis* (New York: A. Philip Randolph Educational Fund, 1967).

4. Quoted by Wilbur H. Ferry in "Must We Rewrite the Constitution to Control Technology?", *Saturday Review,* March 2, 1968, p. 53.

Comment

William L. Kissick

In developing my comments on Professor Somers' discussion I have decided to grasp the nettle by hazarding some guesses as to where I think we might be going.

I would agree with most of his statements in the section entitled "Prices, Utilization, and Cost," as well as with those under the heading of "Quality." I think these are fairly accurate observations concerning many of the problems that confront us. I shall focus my remarks on the issues raised under the heading "Delivery of Services and Planning."

The Challenge of Our Time

I think the theme of the challenge presented to our time is set nicely by Gerard Piel when he states (in Chapter 3) that the laissez-faire market process cannot successfully organize the modern technology required for the delivery of comprehensive personal health services. This assumption has become increasingly pervasive and is rapidly approaching the status of conclusion among individuals concerned with the structure and function of the health enterprise. However, I think we have crossed the threshold from a toleration of the chaos so effectively documented by Professor Somers, and have initiated a search for pragmatic solutions to our problems.

Do we know where we are going? In general terms, yes. In my opinion, the direction has been specified by the National Advisory Commission on Health Facilities in its Report to the President dated December, 1968. The chief conclusion: "The nation must concentrate on the organization of health facilities and other resources into effective, efficient and economical community systems of comprehensive health care available to all."[1]

This objective, or some paraphrase of it, is at the center of much of our thinking. What are the implications of this kind of objective? What are the policy choices involved? In trying to develop a few predictions, I offer my impressions of some of the implications of the social policy decisions in effect since 1965, suggest what kinds of pressures they have generated, and posit what some of the axes of solution might be.

Recent Trends in Health Policy

First, in the area of financing, I think that Title XVIII and Title XIX of the Social Security Act of 1965—Medicare and Medicaid—have launched us on a course of action that will result in the attainment of complete coverage of the costs of health care; i.e., universal health insurance. By this I mean that virtually all of the population will be budgeting and prepaying their health care costs. I do not know how long it will take—perhaps a decade or two—but I am convinced we are moving in that direction.

To re-emphasize Gerard Piel's statement already referred to, universal coverage cannot be attained in the uncontrolled market process. If we were to find the resources and pump them into the system, or the "nonsystem," as now constituted, I do not think we could realize universal coverage. How then are we to develop a modified market system? This is the next critical issue. Planning, the last issue to which Professor Somers addresses himself, will be at the center of the developments concerned with the realization of a modified market system. These developments will represent the areas in which efforts are focused on the organization and delivery of services.

As Professor Somers notes, "the Hill-Burton Hospital Survey and Construction Act of 1946 was the nation's first significant instrumentality for a limited form of planning." I would add that the planning, as suggested by the early reports of Surgeon General Parran's staff, was an idea whose time had not yet come. It was several years in advance of social readiness. This was brought home to me significantly when I read Stephen Bailey's *Congress Writes A Law,* a discussion of the Congressional battles around the Full Employment Act of 1946.[2] It emerged, as you know, as the Employment Act of 1946; "full" was conspicuously missing from the title.

As Bailey assessed the mood of Congress and the deliberations around this particular piece of legislation, he suggested that one of the reasons Congress passed it, and authorized the establishment of the Council of Economic Advisors responsible to the President, is that most Congressmen were convinced that no President in his right mind would indeed try to plan for the economy; therefore, it seemed relatively safe and innocuous to authorize him to do so.

I think Bailey was fairly accurate in his prediction, at least for about the first ten to fifteen years in the life of the Council of Economic Advisors. However, the time was not wasted, as it was spent in developing methodology, a data base, and so forth. It was not until Walter Heller came to Washington as Chairman of the Council of Economic Advisors in the Kennedy Administration that some of the fuller implications of the Employment Act were realized.[3]

In my opinion, the 1960's brought the recognition that, for the health enterprise, planning is imperative. Although imperative, the questions remain: How and to what end? What are the alternatives? These are among the foremost questions at the present time. Professor Somers has suggested the general magnitude of the alternatives. For me, the alternatives are analogous to an assessment of the issues by Theodore Vail when he was appointed President of the Bell Telephone System during the first decade of this century. His analysis led him to conclude that the alternatives were either a strongly regulated public utility or a nationalized phone service. This did not meet with much approval from his Board of Directors. Vail was fired, only to be rehired when the directors became even more alarmed over the public demand for nationalization of the telephone than they were over Vail's advocacy of public regulation.[4]

I think that we are at a comparable crossroads in health at the present time. The issues are those of *institutionalization* and *accountability* in the delivery of health services. If one were to present social action on a scale extending from absolute free enterprise at one extreme to total public endeavor on the other, health would occupy a position closer to the free enterprise pole. Health services for medical care have never occupied the extreme position of free enterprise, however. Restrictions of licensure, certification, and accreditation have served to establish standards and constraints that are in the public interest.

In the evolution of the quest for health from an ecclesiastical endeavor to a community enterprise, there has been a search for the appropriate context and structure in which to vest authority for allocation of resources. I think that search is now probably the most intense it has ever been, and will probably be at the very center of the developments over the years and decades ahead.

The principal issue in health at the present exists in attempts to define a middle-ground position of community responsibility that merges private initiative and public accountability. We are searching for a social instrument short of government that functions adequately in the public interest. Perhaps a social utility, to use the terms of Eveline Burns in her excellent postscript to the Piel Commission report;[5] or a quasi nongovernmental organization—the kind of instrumentality suggested by Alan Pifer of the Carnegie Corporation in his 1968 annual report;[6] or a franchised service not unlike the airlines, with governmental regulation and standards—the concept espoused by Kerr White in a paper presented to the American Association for the Advancement of Science in 1967.[7]

This, in my opinion, is what Regional Medical Programs (RMP)—or the Heart Disease, Cancer, and Stroke Amendments of 1965—and the comprehensive health planning and public health service amendments of 1966 (Public Law 89-749) are all about. We have launched two massive social experiments in search of the optimal answers. To date, as Professor Somers notes, there is a paucity of scholarship concerning the health enterprise. I could not agree with him more. The problems are evident (a fairly recent issue of *Time*[8] has certified this for us so that we now know for certain they exist); but what are the answers?

Health Services Technostructures

RMP, in my opinion, is an attempt to realize through regionalization the health version of John Kenneth Galbraith's "technostructure," as described in *The New Industrial State.*[9] Public Law 89-749, a partnership for health, is a pursuit, somewhat confusing and random at times but a pursuit nonetheless, of the "institutional infrastructure of modern organized society" discussed by Gunnar Myrdal in his essays *Beyond the Welfare State.*[10]

Let me elaborate on the specifics of these pursuits to suggest in greater detail some of the ideas I have in mind. In RMP there is an effort to bring about a relationship referred to as cooperative arrangements among and between institutions—a very tenuous courtship. I doubt that at the present time the institutions are even up to the stage of holding hands, let alone embracing or keeping company with each other; but I suspect there will be a sequence of relationships that become more intimate and interdependent. I think the forces that will bring this about are suggested by Gerard Piel in Chapter 3. Technology, as well as the demand for services, will force this institutional interdependency, their collaboration, and then ultimately, I think, contractual relationships—even mergers.

Chapter 2 of Galbraith's *The New Industrial State* is addressed to the "Imperatives of Technology." I shall quote a few paragraphs, adding some comments as I go along.

> Technology's most important consequence . . . is in forcing the division and subdivision of any task into its component parts. Thus and only thus can organized knowledge be brought to bear on performance . . . It can only be applied if the task is so subdivided that it begins to be coterminous with some established area of scientific and engineering knowledge.

Substitute "medical" for "engineering," and the comparison is very nicely made.

> Nearly all of the consequences of technology derive from this need to divide and subdivide tasks, to bring knowledge to bear on these functions, and to combine the finished elements into a whole.

Adapting Galbraith's statement to health, the finished elements are combined into some comprehensive array of services (rather than an industrial product).

Galbraith posits the following six consequences of technology:

> 1. An increasing span of time separates the beginning from the completion of any task.

This is, I think, most nicely demonstrated for us in the space program. The objective was set in 1961, to be realized only in 1969 when an astronaut did indeed take a stroll on the lunar surface.

2. There is an increase in the capital that is committed ... The increased time, and ... the increased investment in goods in process cost money. So does the knowledge that is applied to the various elements of the task.

This knowledge is extraordinarily complex and costly. More than two and a half billion dollars are being spent annually for biomedical and health-related research. As large as this investment is, it is small in comparison to the enterprise it sustains. In-house staff analysis by the Office of Science and Technology revealed that technologically dependent growth industries in the late 1950's and early 1960's were investing approximately 10 per cent of their gross income in research and development.[11] A comparable investment by the nation's health enterprise about 1975 with projected gross expenditures in excess of $100 billion would be $10 billion, of a four-fold increase over present levels. As we compare investment needs of the above magnitude with the relatively small capital base of the individual components of the health enterprise, I think we can appreciate the forces that will foster institutional collaboration leading to corporate mergers.

3. With increasing technology the commitment of time and money tends to be made ever more inflexible to the performance of a particular task. That task must be precisely defined before it is divided and subdivided into its component parts ... If that task is changed new knowledge and new equipment will have to be brought to bear.

Many of the problems—and they are costly problems indeed—associated with current efforts to develop hospital information systems (HIS) are a consequence of the difficulties with definition and with specification of performance criteria. Physicians, nurses, and other professional and technical health manpower resist standardization of their communication even though it is critical to accurate and reproducible transmission of information among and between an increasing number of users. Add to this the proclivity of the numerous individual practitioners in the institutional subsystem to modify their "art form" almost at will, and one can appreciate the awesome challenge by and to technology. The level of investment required is suggested by the experience of American Airlines and International Business Machines. The development of SABRE, the passage reservation system, took some five years and cost in excess of $50 million. Moreover, the specifications are simple in comparison to those for a medical record system or a hospital information system.[12]

4. Technology requires specialized manpower.

We have specialized, if not over-specialized, manpower. This brings me to the fifth point made by Galbraith:

5. The inevitable counterpart of specialization is organization ... that brings the work of specialists to a coherent result. If there are many

specialists this coordination will be a major task ... massive and complex organizations are the intangible manifestations of advanced technology.

Organization is one of the missing elements in the current health enterprise. It is certain to be the foremost task ahead.

6. From the time and capital that must be committed, the inflexibility of the commitment, the needs of large organization and the problems of market performance under conditions of advanced technology comes the necessity for planning.

Planning becomes the imperative. The analogy may not be completely appropriate, but I think that RMP provides the opportunity to formulate the health services equivalent of Galbraith's "technostructure."

We have a suggestion of the precursor in the Kaiser Foundation medical care plan.[13] I suspect that insurance companies, when they start buying hospitals and employing doctors, will launch us on the way to organizing health care corporations, social utilities, or franchised services. In so doing, would it be unreasonable to expect the Blue Cross plans of the nation to become solely consumer-dominated, and thus to realize the benefits of two-party bargaining, negotiation, and contractual relationships, in lieu of the anomalous third-party situation that exists at the present time? In the current third-party situation, the Blues are neither a party of the first nor a party of the second part.

The Institutional Infrastructure of Health Care

The desire to retrieve the consumer bargaining power dissipated through third-party vendors has led to the organization of the California Council for Health Plan Alternatives "to seek a fundamental reorganization of health care." A statement by its chairman, Einar O. Mohn, who is also Director of the Western Conference of Teamsters, recalls a statement by Gerard Piel; Mohn said that "the real crisis is that the billions being poured into health care actually are feeding the inflationary fires and providing very little incentive to find more effective ways of organizing and delivering health services."[14] Further on in the same address Mohn warns that "It would be wise for hospitals to recognize that the days are limited when they will be able to increase rates without being accountable to the public." What is accountability? I have spoken only to the institutional relationships that could come to grips with some of the problems of organizing and delivering health services. The California Council for Health Plan Alternatives seeks "accountability" by pooling "the collective bargaining power of a million and three-quarters organized workers." What are some alternatives? This brings me to Public Law 89-749.

Much of the confusion surrounding this law results from the fact that it is a combination of two pieces of legislation, one dealing with planning and the other with grants. The first three sections (A, B, and C) concern themselves with planning, that is, the effort to develop the planning competency and a planning base, at the state level (A), at the local or area-wide level, recognizing the necessity for overlapping political jurisdictions (B), and at the level of investing in the development of health planning competency (C). The last two sections (D and E) are an effort to pursue on a small scale an implementation of the Heller proposals for block grants to the states, as a substitute for categorical grants.

The first three sections are addressed conceptually to the issue of the "institutional infrastructure of organized society," discussed by Myrdal. To quote from his essay:

> The whole character of our national communities is changing . . . public policy is now decided upon and executed in many different sectors and on different levels . . . by the central state . . . provincial and municipal authorities . . . by a whole array of "private" power groups organized to promote group interests and common causes . . .
>
> Within the framework of state controls, the organizations have gained and not lost in influence . . . regulatory coordination undertaken by state authorities is ordinarily carried out only after consultation and actually in cooperation with the organizations . . . the increasing strength, number and activity of the organizations . . . has meant a spreading out of participation, initiative and influence . . . to ever larger sections of the people . . . it represents a decentralization of the making and implementation of public policies.[15]

This is the gamble of Public Law 89-749. When the legislation was passed, there were clearly a few strong vested interests in the health enterprise. No single interest can move beyond some state of being vested with less than a comprehensive view of the problem. Can other vested interests emerge? The law acknowledges that health is too important to be left to health professionals. The issue is thrown open to a larger array of vested interests in the hope that countervailing powers will emerge to address the problems. In a sense, the California Council for Health Plan Alternatives suggests that the gamble will pay off.

But what of other approaches to accountability? Is franchising pursued in New York State under the Folsom Act the answer?[16] Is the approach in Rhode Island, a uniform reporting system emphasizing full disclosure of information on performance, attempted measures of quality, and the yield of services for investments and operating costs, to be preferred?[17] I do not know the answer, and I have yet to be very much convinced by anybody who thinks he does. I do not think we have the data base, the methodology, or the experience at the present time to formulate an argument that goes beyond polemic for the most viable answers.

The Future Agenda

As we develop the competencies, methodology, and data base of social economics, I think we will be able to realize for the health care economy that circumstance sought by the late President Kennedy in his Commencement Address at Yale University in 1962. He said: "What is at stake in our economic decisions today is not some grand warfare of rival ideologies which will sweep the country with passion, but the practical management of a modern economy."[18]

Professor Somers' concluding remarks bear repeating; it is indeed commonplace to read in the health care literature the familiar warning to different components of the industry that if they do not start to move in the right direction the government may take over. Hypothetically, just what would the government do if it should take over? Short of nationalization and subcontracting with the Department of Defense, I do not know. With Professor Somers, I must ask whether we know what we would want it to do. I agree most emphatically that perhaps, if we did, we could find more effective means for our goals than such a takeover. For me this seeking for means is what the Institute for Social Economics at Temple University and The Leonard Davis Institute for Health Economics at the University of Pennsylvania are all about: The issues are there; the answers must be found.

Notes

1. U.S. National Advisory Commission on Health Facilities, *Report to the President* (U.S. Government Printing Office, 1968).

2. Stephen K. Bailey, *Congress Writes A Law* (New York: Columbia University Press, 1950).

3. Walter W. Heller, *New Dimensions in Political Economy* (Cambridge: Harvard University Press, 1966).

4. Peter F. Drucker, *The Effective Executive* (New York: Harper and Row, 1967).

5. Eveline M. Burns, "The Challenge and The Potential of The Future," in *Comprehensive Community Health Services in New York City,* Report of the Commission on the Delivery of Personal Health Services (New York, 1968).

6. Alan Pifer, "The Quasi-Non-Governmental Organization," in *Annual Report of the Carnegie Corporation of New York* (1968).

7. Kerr, White, "Personal Incentives, Professional Standards and Public Accountability in the Provision of Personal Health Services," paper presented before 134th Meeting, American Association for the Advancement of Science (New York: 1967).

8. "What's Wrong With American Medicine?", *Time* 93:53-58 (February 21, 1969).

9. John K. Galbraith, *The New Industrial State* (Boston: Houghton Mifflin, 1967). All quotations are from Chapter 2.

10. Gunnar Myrdal, *Beyond the Welfare State* (New Haven: Yale University Press, 1960).

11. Jerrold Zacharios, Personnel Communication, Summer Study of Medical Education, Endicott House, Massachusetts (July, 1965).

12. G. Octo Barnett, Presentation to Computer Section, National Institutes of Health, 1967.

13. *Report of the National Advisory Commission on Health Manpower,* op. cit., vol. 2, appendix IV.

14. Einar O. Mohn, "What to Do About Rising Hospital Costs" (Burlingame, California: California Council for Health Plan Alternatives, 1968).

15. Myrdal, op. cit.

16. New York Public Health Law, Article 28.

17. Rhode Island Public Laws, Ch. 171, amending Chapter 23-16, General Laws of Rhode Island.

18. John F. Kennedy, Commencement Address, Yale University, 1962, in *Public Papers of the Presidents: John F. Kennedy, 1962* (Washington: U.S. Government Printing Office, 1963), pp. 470-475.

Comment

Nelson H. Cruikshank

I am very happy to have the privilege to make some comments on Dr. Somers' discussion. It is provocative, as he meant it to be, and it is, by design, negative in impact and emphasis, presenting some well-defined and documented problems.

Wage Increases and Hospital Costs

First of all, I want to document Dr. Somers' remark that the spiraling costs of care have been more profound than the recent wave of hospital wage increases, which seems to be the current favorite scapegoat.

I suppose I hear more about this than some others. When I complain about the rising cost of hospital care, and about the spiraling fees for medical services, my friends say, "Well, Nelson, if you will just call off your boys from asking for wage increases we can hold these costs down"—as if I had the authority or power to call them off (some people have peculiar ideas about the labor movement).

It is always presented as a kind of challenge to me—that rising hospital costs are a direct result of rising wages. Based on figures from the Department of Health, Education and Welfare, I do not think this argument holds.

Table 1 contains, with respect to hospitals, information on hospital expenses, year by year. The first column, on payroll as a per cent of total expense, shows that in the period from 1960 to 1968, payroll as a per cent of total expense went down from 62.3 per cent to 59.6 per cent. That is not much of a decrease, but it gives the lie to the charge that the payroll expense is the main cause of increases in hospital costs.

The second column shows the percentage of annual increase in payroll expense. The low is 9.6 per cent in 1965; the increase jumped to 11.2 per cent in 1966 and to 16.5 per cent in 1968. But it is not quite as horrendous as it would appear to be, particularly in view of the fact that the percentage increase in expenses other than payroll ranged to 20.9 per cent (in the year 1967; see the third column). This is significant and probably when viewed in relation to the figures in the first column, accounts for more of the rise in hospital expenses than do wages.

Concealed within these general figures are other important facts. Take payroll expense itself. This includes a lot of payrollees who are not the people in unions pressing for increases. They are not the charwomen and the low-paid custodial people that have been at last coming into their own in the wage structure. It includes some of the better-paid subprofessionals.

TABLE 1

Payroll and Other Expenses of
Non-Federal Short-Term General
Hospitals, 1960-1968

Year	Payrolls as % of Total Expense	Annual Increase in Payroll Expense (%)	Increase in Non-Payroll Expense (%)[a]
1960	62.3	10.6	9.9
1961	61.6	10.0	13.4
1962	61.9	10.0	8.6
1963	61.7	9.8	10.6
1964	61.7	10.8	10.8
1965	61.7	9.6	9.5
1966	61.1	11.2	14.2
1967	60.0	15.4	20.9
1968	59.6	16.5	18.2

[a]Equipment, services, expansion of services, etc.

Source: *Journal of the American Hospital Association,* "Guide Issues,"
August 1, 1964, 1967, and 1969.

TABLE 2

Average Annual Percent Increases
in Hospital Daily Service Charges,
CPI, Selected Periods, 1960-1969

Period	Increase (%)
1960-65	6.3
1965-66	9.6
1966-67	19.1
1967-68	13.2
1968-69	13.0

Source: Consumer Price Index, Bureau of Labor Statistics, U. S. Department
of Labor.

Table 2 shows that with regard to the hospital daily service charges, the average increase in the years 1960-65 was 6.3 per cent. In 1966-67 it went up to 19.1 per cent; it fell back in 1967-68 to 13.2 per cent, and in 1968-69 to 13.0 per cent. But, of course, that is 13.0 per cent on this increased base, so in absolute amounts it is not a great deal less than the increase in the year before.

One other comment about this wage issue, without belaboring it too much: As Gerard Piel notes, there was a kind of involuntary philanthropy on the part of the low-paid worker prior to the time he began to press for the higher wages. The matter is complicated further by the fact that there were concealed costs; that is, there were costs of hospitals that did not show up in the daily charges and these costs were borne by the very large subsidy derived from the substandard wages paid to hospital workers.

Also, the wage increases which are being talked about so much and are used as a kind of rationale for the rapid increase in costs, particularly for hospitals, have not been great. In 1967 the Fair Labor Standards Act first became applicable to hospitals and it gave a special rate to hospitals in recognition of the very low wages that had been paid in the past. In 1967, for example, the minimum wage applicable to hospitals was $1.00 an hour. In 1968 it was raised to $1.15 an hour, which was $.45 an hour below the minimum wage applicable in other activities. This was a recognition on the part of Congress that hospital wages started from an extraordinarily low base. In 1969, the hourly minimum wage for hospitals became $1.30; for a person working forty hours a week, this rate works out to an annual income of only $2,600, which is still below the poverty level. No person working at the legal minimum wage in a hospital today can support a family.

So wages are not so high in hospitals, to begin with, and the increases have not been so startling as some defenders of the system would claim. In 1966, the last year for which wage data of this kind were available, only about a third (34.3 per cent) of the employees starting from this very low base received as much as a 10 per cent increase, and only 7.6 per cent received an increase of as much as 20 per cent.

These figures need to be borne in mind when some hospital administrators tell us that these "tremendous" increases in wage costs are the main cause of rising hospital costs.

This is something of a side point and I certainly do not argue against Dr. Somers' main conclusion, that there is little doubt of the validity of these general trends. Certainly costs are going up, but the facts do not support the claim that rising hospital costs are mainly a result of the long-delayed application of justice to hospital wage scales.

Dr. Somers uses several quotations that make good source materials; but it seems to me that he has not drawn from them exactly the right conclusions; at any rate, he has not drawn the same conclusions I have.

Raising Productivity in the Health Industry

Dr. Somers quotes John Dunlop's statement, "The permanent problem is the need for more productivity." I certainly agree, but I would point out that to a large degree, this is what distinguishes this economic activity from other more characteristically economic activities in our country. Looking at the history of the growth and development of economic activity in this country, it can be described, with the dangers attendant on all generalizations, as the product of two pressures: the upward pressure of manpower shortages and the downward pressure of a competitive situation.

For a long time the frontier situation drained off our surpluses; the productive scheme was developed in the shadow of a manpower shortage, or at least of a potential manpower shortage, because in periods of high unemployment the frontier was there to drain off the surpluses. This is in contrast to the general situation in Europe. When the frontier was gone, and when the artificial pump-priming was discontinued, after World War I, the labor movement at last developed to the point at which its demands in collective bargaining substituted for the manpower shortage and did something to control the labor market.

Surely we have some combines and certain strong tendencies toward monopoly, but nothing like those that exist in the cartel system in Europe. Generally our system can be characterized as a competitive one. While I give due credit to the ingenuity of American management, I do not think our managers are really any smarter than European management. Rather, I believe that the pressure of labor demands and the shortage of labor, even though it may be artificially created by the unions controlling manpower supplies and rates in a competitive situation is what has forced management in this country to be extraordinarily ingenious in developing efficient methods that have increased output.

What is lacking, in part, in the health system is that neither of these factors has been present. The health system has operated virtually outside the dynamics of the American productive system. I know there are weaknesses in any analogy, particularly in this field; but, as a contrast, let us take the automobile industry. I remember very well that in 1912 my father purchased a Buick and paid $1,100 for it. Adjusted for price increases in manufactured goods, that sum is equal to about $3,190. Wage rates in the manufacturing industry in 1912 were $.21 an hour. At the end of 1968 they were a little over $3.00 an hour (this is in general manufacturing; rates were a little higher in the automobile industry). This is close to a 1,500 per cent increase in wages. But at the end of the 1960's a basic Buick, which is a better automobile than the 1912 Buick, cost about $2,500. If one adjusts for price differentials, this is only $500 more. In absolute dollars, the price of Buicks has increased about 220 per cent, while the wages have increased 1500 per cent.

How can an industry increase its wage rates fifteen times and the price of its product by only two times, or a little over two times? It does so by rationalization, dynamic enterprise, imagination, and efficiency that increases productivity.

I know that the hospital industry and the health industry are service industries and that service industries are not comparable in many respects to manufacturing enterprises but there are some things that service industries can learn from manufacturers and industrial management. The men in charge of the health enterprise should be inquiring all along the line about what can be learned. The Kaiser plan has shown, in the construction, design, and management of hospitals, for example, that management efficiency, utilization of manpower, better design of equipment, and many managerial practices can be borrowed from industrial experience and applied in the health field.

Attitudes Toward "Government Money" and the Concept of Insurance

Professor Somers hints at a solution in the matter of costs but does not make any specific proposals. He refers to the advantages of grants as against loans in the matter of capital cost and then condemns the practice of allowing each hospital to be the sole judge of its own capital needs, which then becomes a tax on the entire community. He points out that this is still the prevailing practice despite all the talk about planning. He mentions that all three of the proposals for meeting capital needs have what he calls the disadvantages of reducing the traditional dependence of hospitals on fund-raising through community participation, giving the population to be served the opportunity to give or withhold approval of hospital policy.

I agree with this completely, but I point out that it is simply a reflection of the new attitude of many hospitals and hospital managers toward what they think of as "government money." It is the easy source of funds now—apparently easier to get than the money of friends and philanthropists—so why not use it, not only to meet the current costs of providing care, but for capital equipment?

This attitude was clearly reflected in the hospitals' requests, which became more nearly demands as they went to Congress and got the Health Insurance Benefits Council and the administration overruled, for a cost reimbursement formula under Medicare.

This, in turn, relates to a point that I shall return to—the insurance concept. It has major weaknesses in our approach to the whole problem with which we are dealing, but it has some advantages too. I shall talk about the weaknesses later. As for advantages, at this stage it is a useful device for reminding hospitals and their spokesmen that Medicare attempts only to set up a mechanism for insuring people against the risk of certain medical bills incurred under the existing medical system and in existing institutions.

The capital costs for these institutions, then, are quite properly a responsibility of the larger community and are not a proper charge against the insurance system. Thus they are not properly a part of the social insurance premium, i.e., the social security taxes payable under Part A of Medicare.

Professor Somers speaks about the deficiencies of Part B, the medical services part of the Medicare program, and the lack of standards for physician services. He gives us an illustration of a certain hospital owned by four physicians and decries the fact, quite properly, that the Medicare law gives the administration authority to stop reimbursement for services in that hospital but not the authority to stop reimbursement to the same doctors for the services they give out of the hospital because these physicians are licensed by the state in which they practice.

He might have made the illustration more striking by pointing out that these doctors have had their licenses suspended, but under the rule of the state in which they live and practice a doctor whose license is suspended and under appeal can still continue to practice, and no one has authority under Medicare to stop payment to them even under such extreme circumstances.

Beyond this, and I think much more significant than this, is that from Professor Somers' remarks the proper conclusion can be drawn that the insurance mechanism is both an inadequate and an inappropriate mechanism for financing health care. Some of those who have followed my arguments in the past may be surprised that I say that. I think it is true for a number of reasons, among them the fact that the insurance mechanism almost obviates the use of preventive services and the financing of preventive services and that it perpetuates many of the worst features of our present medical care system.

Recently, at one of those gatherings sponsored by The Brookings Institution (where doctors are brought together in very comfortable surroundings so they can feel perfectly at home), I shared a panel position with a former official of the American Medical Association. I said to him, "You know, we were both on the wrong side of the barricades in the fight over Medicare." You remember the arguments: The AMA went to great lengths to try to convince the public and Congress that social security is not insurance and that therefore Medicare, if it ever passed, would not be insurance; that it was a welfare program, tax supported, and so forth, and could not properly be called insurance. I said to him, "You should have attacked the Medicare proposal on the ground that it *was* insurance rather than health planning and health financing, and then you would have been on your own ground and you might have won. Also, you might have had us on the other side of the barricades helping you because it was the attitude of the medical profession insisting that social insurance was not insurance, and the attitude they took in other respects, that forced those of us who wanted to take the next step forward to fall back on an existing mechanism that had wide public acceptance and which could be explained to Congress."

I think if the consumer groups and the medical profession had been able to combine and say "Just making money available is not all that's needed for good health. We need something different from the present health care system in America," with the prestige and the acceptance and the credibility that attaches to the medical profession on Capitol Hill we could have sold an entirely different kind of program. But since there was no such combination, and the position of the AMA was one of rigid, inflexible opposition to any change, we were forced to use the awkward and inadequate approach of an insurance mechanism.

In Defense of Medicare

Having criticized Medicare on this ground, I would like to point out several things, drawing on what I think is documentation for my conclusions in Dr. Somers' presentation even though he does not quite draw these conclusions.

There are some things that I think need to be said in defense of Medicare, particularly since Gerard Piel is quite critical of it. In my view and in the view of a great many supporters of Medicare, it is a transitional stage. It was the next possible step. It was not the ideal. We knew there were some things wrong about it when we were carrying it forward, but it was the only possible next step that could be taken at the time because of the public's level of understanding of the nature of the health problem. People were still thinking in terms of the accessibility problem and of removing the economic barrier.

Of course, the accessibility problem was particularly acute for older people because they had been largely left out of the expanding services of private insurance, both the commercial and the Blue Cross and Blue Shield.

Secondly, it is true that there are some faults and weaknesses in the Medicare system and that these are imbedded in Medicare, but it is also true that these weaknesses and shortcomings are now more visible and have been made more visible by the fact of Medicare than they ever were before.

This is partly a result of my third point: When faced with the problem of how to bring about legislative change or any change that one wants to make, one has to take into account the feelings, the attitudes, the traditions, and the mores of people at a given moment in time, and one has to build on them if possible.

People in America are traditionally more critical of a program in which public money is spent and in which the government is involved than they are of private enterprises doing exactly the same thing. It is a theory of mine that people in America have a way of getting mad at what they are told to get mad at. If the government treated them as the Pennsylvania Railroad treats its passengers, for example, there would be a revolution, but nobody tells people to get mad at the Pennsylvania Railroad. People are told, however, in editorials, and in editorialized news treatments, to get mad at the government.

In a way this is good. Its roots go back to the Jeffersonian tradition of being critical and skeptical of government. But with respect to Medicare, I think, one can say categorically that everything wrong in Medicare was also and to a greater degree wrong in Blue Cross, Blue Shield, and private health insurance, but that what people tolerated easily in the private insurance approach they will be very critical of in government.

To the extent that we have moved the program out of the private area we have not really created these evils, weaknesses, or faults. All we have done is make them visible and, hence, vulnerable. Happily, there is thus a better chance to overcome them in a government program than there is in a private program.

Beyond the Insurance Principle in Health Care

Professor Somers, in my view, supports the conclusion that we must move from the concept of insurance to the concept of community planning for health care; and that is a great change. He says that in no other realm of economic life are payments guaranteed for costs that are neither controlled by competition nor regulated by public authority, and in which no incentives for economy can be discerned. I agree; I cannot quarrel with the statement, except to point out (going further than Dr. Somers does in my conclusion) that under Medicare the government is not really purchasing medical care. He does not say this, but I like to point out that in this particular aspect of our system we are really insuring the covered individual against the contingency of a medical bill.

The cost-reimbursement formula in Medicare is only a mechanism for determining the degree of risk to which the insured is exposed. This is not a defense of Medicare. I only point out that this approach has inherent in it the factors that lead to many of the problems which Dr. Somers and others have emphasized.

Professor Somers quotes from a provocative paper by the economist Victor Fuchs and draws the conclusion that our well-advertised magnificent resources are distributed very inequitably, that the country has both excellent and very poor quality of care. I agree, but I think there is something even more significant in what Fuchs had to say; namely, the conclusion that our medical resources have been distributed not on the basis of health needs at all, but on the basis of effective market demand.

If we were to array all of society's possible options in distributing resources for medical care, ability to pay for care is the worst possible option. But that is the one we have selected, that is the basis on which we make both the geographical distribution and other kinds of allocations of medical services and facilities. I think this only illustrates Gerard Piel's point: the market mechanism is inadequate to meet this problem.

This too points to the essence of the argument about whether medical care is a right or a privilege. When Dr. Rouse, an AMA president, objected to the statement that medical care is a right he was defending the old position that medical care is indeed a privilege and should be available on the basis of the individual's ability to pay for it, as Cadillacs are. You don't find many Cadillac agencies in the ghetto, and you don't find much health service either, aside from some charity medium.

What we should really be asking is whether the practice of medicine and the delivery of health services is indeed an appropriate area for free enterprise. Anyone who thinks this is not a real question has been reading the *AMA Journal* and the *New England Journal of Medicine*. If he read *Medical Economics* or, more especially, the *AMA News,* he would find it to be a very real question.

Money, Manpower, and Motivations

Dr. Somers raises the question whether simply expending more money will solve the problem of meeting the needs of the poor. He implies a negative answer, and I agree; but this also points to the need for physicians and others in the whole medical setup with basically different motivations. I offer this conclusion realizing that it may present an even bigger problem than the one we have, but I think we have got to grasp the nettle. There is something fundamentally wrong about the basic motivation and setup of our whole system.

Somers and many others are quite properly pointing out that the problem rests in the structure and organization of our medical care system, but I think this is only part of the truth and I am not sure it is the most important part. The medical care "system" is perfectly structured to do what it is meant to do, namely, to make money for private practitioners. So, gauged by what it sets out to do, it does a magnificent job. To this end, manpower is properly limited to meet the demands of the customers who can afford to pay. We have, of course, many fine hospitals under the direction of many highly motivated individuals and administrators, but there are also many, many hospitals which are simply workshops financed by charitable drives, public taxes, and insurance premiums for entrepreneurs who have an M. D. degree in order that they can make money at the expense of the help. That is the driving motivation of much of our health enterprise, and until that motivation is changed we will not change the structure.

These purposes have been misdirected to a large degree. When we begin to dedicate our energies and our organizational abilities to meeting the health needs of the people as we find them, on the basis of analysis and study, then the structure will be easier to change. But I do not think we are going to go about it by tinkering with machinery and structure and ignoring the problem of motivation. As long as our equipment is set up to make money for the private entrepreneurs in the health field, we will have this awkward, inadequate, and inappropriate structure; but if we set ourselves different goals, I believe the restructuring will come with relative (but only relative) ease.

If I were asked how we can accomplish this enormous change, I would answer this way: The leaders of thought, the community leaders, and those in the profession will have to face up to the issue, and if I have properly put my finger on a basic cause the first thing to do is to admit that cause, admit that there is something wrong about the concepts of free enterprise and private profit in health care. This will be an ideological change that will be very difficult to accept.

The second step is a process of educating the public and educating those in the health field to change their attitudes. I describe education (because it will be adult education, largely) as the interpretation of experience. All the things that are happening under Medicare and all the things that are happening under the health planning laws and schemes, the deficiencies which Dr. Somers puts his finger on—all these things are going to be a part of the education. We are in a transitional stage. People in university centers, for instance, will have to interpret to others, and this interpretation of experience is the essence of the health education most needed now.

The third step goes beyond gentle persuasion; it will take a little muscle. By the collective effort of all of us in our various capacities—by reshaping collective bargaining plans (and labor has contributed to all of these faults through the kinds of things we in labor have helped perpetuate under our collective bargaining health plans), by using cooperatives, and by working through the government—we will use our economic muscle in a collective form, as consumers acting together, to balance what has heretofore been the virtually undisputed and unchallenged position of control and power of the provider of medical care, namely, the doctor.

As a former merchant seaman, and an amateur sailor, I have been drawn to read Admiral Morison's history of navigation, which has a very interesting section dealing with the basis of the authority of the sea captain. The author asks himself this question: How can it be that one man in charge of a ship far away from the protection of law, out on the lonely ocean—one man alone in authority over a crew of perhaps forty or fifty men—can order his crew to go into continuing danger, into activities that mean continuing hardship, and yet be virtually certain that although the crew outnumbers him and could overpower him physically at any moment, there will be no mutiny? Morison explains that on the lonely high seas the captain was the only man who could take the chart out of the rack, spread it out, and put his finger down and say, "We are there." Because he was the only one with that special knowledge, he was the only one who knew how to get back to home port. He was God, he was law, he was all power and unquestionable authority on the vessel. That has been the position of the doctor to date, and in Medicare, in effect, the doctors of America have said, "Well, you licked us in the halls of Congress, but you can't run this program without us and you're going to run it on our terms." So far they have, by and large, gotten away with it, but I don't think this situation will prevail for long. Consumers are organizing. They are becoming better informed. They are becoming more aware. Government is going to respond to the pressures of the public against ever-spiraling costs by saying, "Just a minute, Doctor. We recognize your professional expertise. We recognize that you are the authority in medical matters. But you're also dealing in matters of economics; these things too affect the lives of people, and we too know something about them. Let's sit down together across the table and bargain with each other."

This is going to be a part of the process, and in doing it I think the medical profession will adjust itself to a new social situation. There will be a sharing and we will be able to move from the limited confines of an insurance concept and an indemnity for the cost of care to broad community planning for health care.

7

Manpower Programs Under New Management: Some Lessons Learned and Their Applications

Sar A. Levitan

Manpower programs have become an integral part of economic policy and welfare programs since the beginning of the 1960's. New manpower programs have been introduced, focusing on the needs of the poorly educated, the unskilled, and the unemployed; and new services have been initiated with varying degrees of success.[1] Over-all expenditures on manpower programs have increased about fifteenfold in one decade, with an outlay of $2.8 billion projected for fiscal 1971 (see Table 3).

Continued growth at these rates and continued experimentation with new manpower programs and services on a broad scale are unlikely in the immediate years ahead. Where the 1960's was a period of expansion and innovation, the next few years are likely to be characterized by more limited growth and by the application of lessons learned from earlier experiments. Barring unforeseen changes in the health of the economy, this maturation of the manpower effort is dictated by several factors.

Determinants in Reshaping Manpower Programs

First, lessons have been learned from the past. While there is no consensus among manpower experts as to the directions of needed changes, there is general agreement about the need to consolidate the categorical programs that have proliferated during recent years. There is clear evidence that varying eligibility criteria, overlapping services, and conflicting regulations have undermined the effectiveness of manpower efforts, and that many

This statement is part of the continuing evaluation of manpower programs conducted by the center for Manpower Policy Studies. The center is funded by a grant from The Ford Foundation.

TABLE 3

Federal Outlays for Manpower Programs,
Fiscal 1961, 1964, 1966-71[a]
(Millions)

	1961	1964	1966	1967	1968	1969	1970	1971
							(estimates)	
Total	$184	$380	$1,346	$1,619	$1,942	$2,011	$2,385	$2,830
Institutional training	—	93	492	566	587	583	658	739
MDTA institutional	—	93	249	221	235	230	233	241
Job Corps	—	—	229	321	299	236	163	175
Concentrated Employment (CEP)	—	—	—	1	25	52	91	103
Work Incentive (WIN)	—	—	—	—	—	28	118	146
Other relief recipients	—	—	13	18	22	34	49	68
O.I.C.	—	—	1	6	5	4	5	5
On-the-job training	—	5	27	53	117	176	280	469
Jobs in the business sector	—	—	—	—	5	46	139	314
MDTA-OJT	—	5	27	53	84	79	74	59
Public service careers	—	—	—	—	13	17	25	51
New careers	—	—	—	—	13	27	34	37
WIN and CEP-OJT	—	—	—	—	3	7	8	9
Work experience and work support	—	—	333	388	504	416	425	458
Neighborhood Youth Corps	—	—	241	253	341	287	312	336
In-school and summer	—	—	178	126	198	182	212	215
Out-of-school	—	—	63	127	143	106	100	121
Concentrated Employment	—	—	—	—	27	56	59	67
Operation mainstream	—	—	10	9	31	37	41	41
Work experience and training	—	—	76	120	98	26	1	—
Foster grandparents	—	—	5	6	8	8	9	9
WIN	—	—	—	—	—	1	3	5
Job placement and support	126	181	276	306	330	344	390	454
Employment service	126	181	262	291	312	317	353	388
CAA outreach	—	—	12	13	16	22	23	23
Child care	—	—	2	2	2	5	14	43
Administration, research, and support	4	17	65	92	108	124	132	157
Administration	4	8	47	56	63	73	75	78
Research	—	2	6	8	9	8	13	24
Experimental and demonstration	—	7	4	19	25	20	20	19
Technical assistance	—	—	1	1	2	10	11	19
Labor market information	—	—	8	8	8	11	11	14
Evaluation	—	—	—	—	1	2	3	4
Vocational rehabilitation	54	84	154	215	297	368	500	553

[a]Includes only outlays by the Departments of Labor and Health, Education, and Welfare.

Note: Details may not add to totals because of rounding.

Source: U.S. Bureau of the Budget.

improvements could be made. Some programs and approaches developed during the 1960's have been clearly ineffective, and resources should be shifted to the more successful efforts.

Second, and more important in determining the cast of manpower efforts in the next few years, is the attitudes and principles of the Nixon administration. President Nixon has consistently supported the idea that the private sector should take a more active role in manpower programs. The ideology of New Federalism is that centralized administration should be reduced and the states' role expanded, and that these functions should be transferred as much as possible from the public to the private sector. Translated into more specific terms, the Republican precepts of the Nixon administration favor incentives for the business sector to hire and train the disadvantaged. On-the-job training is preferred over institutional training, private over public employment programs, and "workfare" over welfare.

The political principles of the Republican administration, combined with a shift in public priorities—e.g., preferring clean air and water over help for the poor—point toward a stabilization of manpower expenditures and indicate a changing emphasis among individual programs. The hope is to increase the effectiveness of manpower programs through operational reorganization.

A caveat is in order. As in the past, the current and projected state of the economy will continue to influence the character of the manpower efforts. Sustained growth will mean that jobs will continue to be generated, even for the unskilled. Manpower programs must then concentrate on matching supply and demand through training and placement efforts and on providing work incentives for those who are employable but not presently in the work force. Manpower programs must also focus on the needs of those who are working full time but at wages so low that they remain in poverty. Inflation exercises pressure on all government programs, and manpower programs have felt the pinch of budgetary constraints. But if the level of unemployment should rise, pressures will develop to expand job creation programs and to provide income maintenance to persons forced into idleness.

The Fiscal 1970 Manpower Budget

The original budget prepared by the Johnson administration for fiscal 1970 showed an increase in aggregate federal manpower outlays. The Nixon administration made some cuts in the total budget and redesigned the structure of several programs. Outlays for manpower programs in 1970 continued to rise, however, as a result of earlier commitments.

The most striking changes during the first year of the Nixon administration indicating program emphasis were the drastic curtailment of the Job Corps and the expansion of Job Opportunities in the Business Sector (JOBS). President Nixon struck out against the costly Job Corps in his 1968 campaign, and most impartial observers of antipoverty programs questioned whether the results, measured by low retention rates and little educational advancement among enrollees, justified the high costs of residency. The administration revamped the program by shifting it from the Office of Economic Opportunity to the Department of Labor, closing the least effective training centers, and opening a few nonresidential centers in cities. There is little question that this was a much needed reform, though the cuts may have been too precipitous to provide alternative programs for the Job Corps clients.

The expansion of funding for the JOBS program, however, was based more on principle than proven effectiveness. (The enthusiasm for the JOBS approach was initially proclaimed by the Johnson administration.)The JOBS program gives subsidies, averaging around $3,000 per slot, to private firms for the hiring and training of disadvantaged workers. By the end of 1969 some 88,000 job placements were claimed under the contract portion of the program, but about three of every five had already terminated. Basic questions remained unanswered about the effectiveness of training offered to enrollees and whether new jobs were really being created for the disadvantaged. Preliminary evidence indicated that in many cases training was meager and that the jobs were little different from those traditionally filled by unskilled and deficiently educated workers. Furthermore, difficulties have been experienced in inducing companies to participate in the contract program. Despite these warning signals, the Nixon administration adopted President Johnson's proposal to nearly triple outlays for JOBS for fiscal 1970 compared with the previous fiscal year. The contract JOBS program did not warrant this emphasis on the basis of proven performance, revealing a strong preference for private-sector involvement on the part of President Johnson and President Nixon. By the end of 1969, the administration was forced to concede that the commitment of funds to JOBS was in excess of need, and the funds allocated to JOBS were curtailed.

Streamlining the Manpower Efforts

Another major development in the manpower field is a bipartisan effort to overhaul and streamline existing manpower programs. Three legislative proposals were put forward in 1969, including one by the administration, which aimed at consolidating and coordinating the categorical and disparate manpower programs.[2] These proposals would bring together the separate programs of the Manpower Development and Training Act and the manpower programs of the Economic Opportunity Act and the Employment Service, insofar as the latter is involved in these programs. Though limited in scope, the administration's proposal, if enacted, would reduce overlapping services and eligibility gaps, and it would permit more individualized treatment, albeit in a limited area. Greater local control is intended, so that these programs can be adapted to local needs.

It is regrettable that the administration's bill did not even include all the programs under the jurisdication of the Labor Department's Manpower Administration. The decision apparently reflected the judgment that a more ambitious scope would weaken the chances of the administration's manpower training bill receiving Congressional approval. But an overhaul of the current manpower programs should recognize the increasing interdependence between public assistance and work-oriented programs and should include the Work Incentive program (WIN), designed to train relief recipients as part of the consolidated manpower package.

The introduction of these manpower bills stems from a common recognition of the need for administrative reorganization. There is little disagreement on this goal. But the three proposals differ in other ways, especially with respect to the responsibilities assigned to federal, state, and local governments. The O'Hara bill, a democratic proposal, would centralize administration in the Department of Labor, and the Steiger bill would transfer authority to state governors. The administration's manpower training bill would pull in states as partners in administering manpower programs without ignoring the responsibilities of elected officials at the local level or the over-all role of the federal government. The bill would bolster the role of state governments; states would receive 75 per cent of the consolidated manpower funds. But there would be a mandatory passing of funds to the larger cities, which would have a right to choose their own prime sponsors for metropolitan manpower programs. The Secretary of Labor would be charged with the responsibility of monitoring federally funded programs to insure that federal objectives are carried out, and the administration's bill would leave the Secretary 20 to 25 per cent of the total manpower funds appropriated by Congress for experimentation and demonstration as well as for initiation of programs where states and localities do not carry out federal objectives.

The bills also place varying stress on the role of public employment, with the administration's bill giving it little attention. These questions obviously have partisan overtones: the Republican bills advocate decentralized administration and de-emphasize public employment, while the Democratic proposal prescribes centralized administration and guaranteed public employment. In the past, manpower legislation has received broad bipartisan support in Congress, and if legislation to consolidate manpower programs is enacted, it would constitute a compromise of the several pending proposals. Insofar as they deal with the management of manpower programs, the administration's proposals are sound and imaginative and should prevail if a nonpartisan atmosphere is achieved. The bill is silent, however, on the commitment of resources.

Workfare and Welfare

A potentially more significant development affecting manpower efforts is President Nixon's Family Assistance Program. Under this welfare proposal, assistance payments would be made to all low-income families with children, including families with a male head who is employed but earning an inadequate income. A family of four with no other income would thus receive a basic annual payment of $1,600; that is, $500 for each of the first two family members and $300 for each additional member.

The manpower aspects of the family assistance proposal focus upon creating work incentives and helping relief recipients find employment. Under this plan, the first $720 of a family's annual income would be disregarded, and benefits would be reduced 50 cents on the dollar for earnings beyond this point. It would provide expanded assistance for day care centers, enabling adults in recipient families to work, and it would provide for remedial training and job placement. In the first year, training and day care expenditures would cost an estimated $600 million of the projected additional total expenditure of $4.4 billion for public assistance.

The manpower components of the family assistance proposal are built on the experience of the Work Incentive program, which was initiated in 1967 to provide work incentives to recipients of Aid to Families with Dependent Children (AFDC). WIN permits the AFDC mother (most AFDC families are headed by a female) to retain the first $30 of her earnings plus one-third of each additional dollar. The program, however, makes little provision for day care and had scant success in finding employment for participants in its training program.

The importance of the Family Assistance Program is not that it liberalizes the work incentives of WIN, an obviously needed improvement, but rather that the proposal would extend these incentives plus the guaranteed income to families with an employed head. It is estimated that the families of the 1.8 million full-time working poor would be covered by the Family Assistance Program.

The Family Assistance Program takes a necessary step toward bridging the gap between welfare and employment. It recognizes the needs of the many who are employed full time but who work at such meager wages that they continue to live in poverty. And it reflects the national ideology and the presidential preference for workfare over welfare in attempting to increase employment among welfare recipients and enabling them to earn as much as possible.

Despite emphasis upon the admirable twofold objective of creating work incentives for those already receiving welfare and providing additional income for the working poor, the Family Assistance Program raises serious dilemmas and falls short on its promises to reduce dependency. The program would increase the number of those working and receiving assistance, and the income supplements might increase reliance upon public assistance as a substitute for wage increases and tend to perpetuate low wage levels as well as irregular and part-time employment. Under this system, two family heads, each with three dependents, could both receive an annual income of $4,000—although one works full time at a rate of $2 per hour and nets $4,000 without benefit of the welfare system, while the other works only half time at the same $2 per hour and makes up the difference with cash supplements, food stamps, and other income in kind available under welfare programs. This system may widen the work choices of low wage earners, but it may also prevent them from ever achieving economic independence.

Judging from the experience of WIN and the work and training efforts of the 1960's, the provision of training through the family assistance program does not necessarily mean that those trained will secure regular employment. Delivery of training to persons in rural areas is costly; many poorly educated and unskilled workers are not motivated to undergo training, and there is no indication that there will be an increase in jobs for them if they undergo successful training. Perhaps most significantly, the program does not contribute to any change in the structure of work and training institutions. A mere transfer of the responsibility for income maintenance from an employer to the federal government without an increase in wage levels will hardly insure decent employment and income for the working poor.

Economic Stabilizer

Possibly the most innovative feature proposed by the administration relating to manpower policy is a trigger mechanism which would increase expenditures for manpower programs when unemployment rises. The goal of this provision of the administration's manpower training bill is to achieve an automatic countercyclical mechanism by increasing expenditures for manpower programs when there is a slack in the economy. Specifically, the administration's manpower training bill proposes an automatic increase of 10 per cent in manpower funds when unemployment reaches 4.5 per cent of the total labor force for three consecutive months.

While this provision attempts to integrate manpower programs with over-all economic policy and is admirable in principle, it is adequate only as an opener. As any poker player knows, more than an initial investment is necessary to win the game, and the soundest economic principles are not good enough to feed unemployed workers and their families. The administration's proposal is only a teaser and needs additional commitment before it becomes part of an effective economic policy. At the FY 1970 level of appropriations, an increase of 10 per cent in funds allocated to the manpower programs covered by the administration's bill means a boost of about $155 million.

The automatic stabilizer proposed by the administration is supposed to compensate the victims of policies aimed at restraining inflation. The additional funds proposed by the administration are adequate to provide only for a small minority of the prospective victims of the constraining economic policies. According to Labor Department estimates, a rise of unemployment from 3.4 per cent (the level of unemployment at the end of 1969) to 4.5 per cent would, during the course of one year, raise the number of persons unemployed 15 weeks or longer from 2.5 million to 3.9 million, and raise the number of persons unemployed 26 weeks or more during the year from 1 million to 1.8 million. More than $2 billion would be required, again using the Labor Department's estimates, to absorb all the long-term unemployed under MDTA or work experience programs.

The resort to temporary countercyclical expenditures to provide income or jobs to the unemployed is not without its precedents. In the 1958-1959 recession, Congress provided for temporary extended unemployment compensation at a total cost of more than $600 million. During 1961-1962, the pricetag of the temporary extended unemployment compensation was nearly $800 million, and an additional $850 million was appropriated to create jobs in depressed areas. It is true that in both cases unemployment rose to 6 per cent and even higher, but our experience during the 1960's clearly indicates that the government should step in before unemployment reaches such a high level. And one of the salutary lessons we have learned from the 1960's is that the threshold of public tolerance for unemployment has declined. The administration's proposal to raise manpower funds when unemployment reaches 4.5 per cent is therefore sound, but it is not commensurate with the needs of those who become victims of governmental fiscal and monetary policies.

The government should assume responsibility for those who become unemployed as a result of its policies to reduce inflationary pressures. Without raising here any questions about the wisdom of these policies, few would argue that the burden of the resulting unemployment should be placed upon those who can least afford it.

Congress would do well to adopt the administration's proposal of automatically boosting the funds allocated to manpower programs by 10 per cent when unemployment reaches 4.5 per cent. But the plan should be extended by boosting manpower funds 10 per cent for each .2 per cent increase in unemployment. This would mean that the funds allocated to manpower programs would rise automatically by 60 per cent ($930 million at FY 1970 level of appropriations) when unemployment reaches 5.5 per cent. This provision, together with another proposal by the administration calling for an automatic extension of unemployment insurance when the number of insured unemployed reaches 4.5 per cent (about equivalent to 5.7 per cent of total unemployment), would provide a measure of automatic aid to the victims of monetary and fiscal policies.

Policy Developments and Directions

From this brief review of the major manpower developments and policies proposed during the first part of the Nixon administration, it would appear that if the administration's programs prevail there will be a leveling off of manpower outlays and a consolidation of individual programs. Some overlap and waste will be eliminated, and the thrust of manpower policy will be to increase the effectiveness of manpower outlays rather than to increase their magnitude. Political forces will·be at work favoring decentralization according to the precepts of the New Federalism, and expanded involvement by the private sector will be stressed. The predicted policy thrusts are necessitated by a combination of economic conditions and political ideology.

The decentralization dictated by the New Federalism concepts can create obstacles to effective administration of federally funded programs. Many states and localities lack the technical and professional manpower needed to administer such programs, and the prevailing low salary scales paid by most states make it unlikely that they will acquire such talent in the near future. While decentralization may lead to decisions more adapted to local needs, it may also result in decisions which contradict national objectives, so that guidelines must be carefully drawn. There must also be explicit recognition of the needs of larger cities, which are often neglected in state programs.

All of these reservations can be overcome by proper design of New Federalism strategies, but they must be given explicit consideration. The administration's manpower training bill provides for the consolidation of manpower programs and deals imaginatively with these problems.

Improved administration alone, however, is not enough to carry out effective programs. It only helps to secure a better return on funds, but it is no substitute for adequate appropriations. During its first year, the Nixon administration stressed economy in manpower programs and avoided making commitments for the expansion of these efforts. This retrenchment dictated by inflationary pressures must remain only temporary. Improving the administration of the manpower programs would also justify, indeed dictate, the expansion of additional funds to meet needs. The National Manpower Policy Task Force put it this way:

> As we enter a new decade, we should take advantage of the lessons that have been learned from the vast experimentation of the sixties. Improving the administration of manpower programs and related services to maximize their impact is just as important at this moment as adding funds, and as the administration of manpower programs is improved, it is essential that funds be further expanded. Considering

the extent of need, the additional funds become even more justifiable as the effectiveness of the programs is enhanced.[3]

Finally, whatever the ultimate fate of the President's family assistance program, it is quite clear that during the years ahead there will be an increasing interdependence between public assistance and work-oriented manpower programs. The family assistance program is an overdue recognition that a full-time job is not necessarily a cure for poverty. Some form of income supplement for the working poor is likely to become widespread in the years ahead. There will also be an increasing need to tie in training programs for relief recipients, along the lines designed by WIN, with those for other persons who experience difficulties in securing and holding a job.

This cursory review of the Nixon administration's record during its first year makes clear that concern about the demise of the Great Society manpower and welfare programs has been exaggerated and premature. The worriers can relax—indications are that the domestic programs inaugurated during the 1960's will continue into the foreseeable future. The administration has begrudgingly given its blessings to the Office of Economic Opportunity and to most manpower efforts initiated in the 1960's. Pronouncements that a better job could be done in administering these measures hardly required great political courage.

The substantive revisions proposed by the Nixon administration will improve the tools in the kit to aid the unskilled, the unemployed, and the poor. However, none of the measures, either singly or jointly, is a substitute for existing programs, and it will take more funds than the administration has been willing to commit to implement the proposals.

Notes

1. Garth L. Mangum, *The Emergence of Manpower Policy* (New York: Holt, Rinehart & Winston, 1969), pp. 35-68.

2. The three major bills introduced in 1969 were Congressman Steiger's Comprehensive Manpower Act (H. R. 10908), Congressman O'Hara's Manpower Act (H. R. 11620), and the administration's Manpower Training Act (H. R. 13472).

3. *Improving the Nation's Manpower Efforts* (Washington: The Task Force, 1970), p. 7.

Comment

Howard Rosen

Is it not too late at this point to offer mere observations and caveats without proposing constructive suggestions to help those who have the very difficult assignment of administering manpower programs? Dr. Levitan is really playing it safe when, after concluding his self-acknowledged "cursory review" of the first year of the Nixon administration, he comes up with the not altogether novel suggestion that more money be spent in carrying out proposals to aid the unskilled, the unemployed, and the poor.

There are these significant areas which Dr. Levitan covers too lightly in his review of manpower programs. He does not explore in any depth the economic stabilizer which provides a trigger mechanism for raising expenditures on manpower programs when unemployment rises. The second subject which is not given much attention is the important issue of integrating manpower programs into economic policy, which flows out of the trigger mechanism concept. The third area which deserved more attention by Dr. Levitan is the family assistance program, which would provide assistance payments to low-income families with children, including families with a male head who is working but not earning an adequate income.

Need for an Early-Warning System

Let us first look at the trigger mechanism concept. A refined trigger mechanism which goes beyond national unemployment statistics, for example, can be used as the long sought early-warning system for identifying specific industries or geographic areas which are experiencing rising unemployment rates. If this economic instrument were sharpened and used properly, we might avoid creating depressed areas, which are so difficult to aid later on. The advantage of the advance warning system would be that attempts could be made to introduce manpower programs at an early stage to reverse unfavorable developments before they have continued for so long that they are no longer amenable to change.

Consideration may also be given to using this mechanism as an anti-inflationary tool in conjunction with the job vacancy data now being collected by the Department of Labor. The trigger concept can be used to react to occupations or skills which are in short supply and contributing to inflationary forces. A trigger reaction can thus be used to initiate, expand, or reduce specific types of manpower programs. If certain occupations are in short supply, or if workers with certain characteristics are being hit harder by loss of jobs than others in the labor force, administrators of manpower programs can offer specific training programs to meet these special problems.

Are Manpower Programs Really an Integral
Part of Our Economic Policy?

Let us turn to the integration of economic policy and manpower programs. Dr. Levitan's first sentence declares that manpower programs have become an integral part of economic policy and welfare programs since the beginning of the 1960's. However, it can be argued that manpower programs have become a part of economic policy but have never been an "integral" part of that policy. Those who take this view compare our active manpower policy with that practiced by the Swedish Labor Market Board, for example, and point out that in Sweden fiscal and monetary policy decisions are made only after full exploration of the manpower implications of these decisions. Thus, changes in interest rates and tax levels—and a host of other economic decisions—are not made until the employment and unemployment impacts are first studied. These same critics assert that we have a long way to go before we can justifiably claim that we have really integrated our manpower and economic policies, citing for example decisions on interest rates made by the U. S. Federal Reserve Board which affect the employment of construction workers. In view of the large concentration of black workers employed as laborers in this industry and the temper of the times, one may indeed wonder whether the decision-makers who called for higher interest rates which would curtail construction activity took into account all the consequences of their policies, notably the risk in unemployment in this industry which was bound to follow.

The same type of question can be raised about the involvement of the officials of manpower programs in fiscal decisions. Because tax decisions affect national economic growth, administrators of manpower programs may have to bear the brunt of possibly training workers for nonexistent jobs. Manpower programs undertaken outside the context of economic policy severely reduce the potential of such programs. I believe that Dr. Levitan is unduly hesitant in stressing this relationship when the Nixon administration has very clearly linked the need for disinflationary economic policy with the need for emphasizing remedial manpower programs.

If the trigger mechanism is built into legislation, decision-makers who, heretofore, have not always demonstrated their sensitivity to the manpower implications of their policies will have to take into consideration the existence of programs which may be stimulated by their decisions. In the long run, the integration effects of bringing together national policies—in the Federal Reserve Board, the Treasury, and the Department of Labor—on a more rational basis may be as important as the programs triggered into action.

Assistance to the Working Poor: Possible
Impact and Research Potentialities

Let me now turn to another area which is touched upon lightly by Dr. Levitan. This is the family assistance program, which has been characterized as one of the most important pieces of social legislation proposed since 1950. This program may have some very significant effects on the mobility patterns of low-income families, the labor-force participation of low-income workers, the supply of workers in low-wage industries, and the minimum wage policies of the country.

To those who have been associated with the development and administration of manpower programs, the family assistance program offers an unusual opportunity to explore many of the issues raised above. Many critics of the manpower programs have complained that administrators have not been able to demonstrate the over-all effectiveness of their programs. Because the government was unable to launch longitudinal studies which would examine the actions of the same workers before, during, and after their exposure to manpower programs, many of the questions heretofore asked of administrators could not be asnwered.

The family assistance program offers an unusual opportunity to establish a before-and-after longitudinal study which could supply meaningful answers to many questions which will, eventually, be raised about the program. If a study were put into effect before the passage of the program—if it passes—a study whereby persons and families who are on welfare could be identified so that their reaction to the family assistance program could be studied, the administrators could be supplied with answers to the questions they will be asked and need to know as program operators.

For example, the administration would want to know whether the establishment of the family assistance program will inhibit the mobility of persons and families on welfare. Will a Negro family of four living in rural Mississippi decide that they can make a go of it there, or will they continue the migratory pattern of moving in stages to large metropolitan centers? Will the labor force participation rate of persons on welfare or low-income employed workers change because of the family income assistance?

Will the family assistance program be a form of subsidy to low-wage employers? Will the supply of workers for low-wage industries be affected by the program? Will the impact of minimum wage laws be affected by providing income assistance to low-wage workers? These are just some of the questions which might be answered intelligently if we identified unemployed and employed persons who might be affected by the introduction of the family assistance program.

The producers of government statistics have been criticized, often quite justly, for providing snapshot, static data which indicate that the subject under study is in trouble. The data do not identify when and why the trouble began. The process of change is too often missing from the information produced. Without this information the timing and location of strategies of intervention too often depend on guestimates.

Longitudinal studies which follow persons during the process of change may offer the possibility of more meaningful answers to complex economic and social problems. Such studies are expensive and slow in yielding insights. This explains why we have seen so few of them. However, if this country is about to launch a multibillion-dollar experiment in income assistance for low-wage workers and job training for welfare recipients, then it would appear incumbent to develop the kind of information that would enable administrators to evaluate the effectiveness of the new family assistance program in comparison with the old welfare program. Longitudinal studies would be a move in the right direction. Without longitudinal studies, crucial decisions may be made affecting millions of people without adequate information for intelligent decision-making.

Comment
Robert A. Levine

The whole is not equal to the sum of its parts. I agree with Sar Levitan's conclusion that the substantive revisions proposed by the Nixon administration in manpower and welfare programs will improve the tools for aiding the unskilled, the unemployed, and the poor, but that none of the measures, either singly or jointly, is a substitute for existing programs, and that it will take more funds than the administration has been willing to commit to implement the proposals. I agree with this conclusion, but on many points I disagree with Dr. Levitan's reasoning; I am inclined to give major credit to the administration where he provides at best faint praise, and to blame where he gives credit.

Income Maintenance Essential to Manpower Development

My major reason for agreement that the administration proposals will indeed improve the tools lies in the proposed family assistance program. Although the administration proposal is not perfect—the Heineman Commission program embodied in proposed legislation by Senator Fred Harris and others would be a substantial improvement—the Nixon plan can still be a major breakthrough in a needed area. Levitan praises the family assistance program lightly and concentrates on its bugs; I would concentrate on the nature of the breakthrough that would occur if the Nixon proposal, the Harris bill, or anything in between were passed. Both proposals provide for the first time, income maintenance for the working poor; a national system of income maintenance administered nationally; built-in incentives for work within the income maintenance system; and a separation of income payments from welfare services. All these changes are badly needed.

More Spending for What?

This breakthrough, to my mind, is the single major relevant and favorable innovation proposed by the Nixon administration in the fields of social welfare. Next to this, even the rising-unemployment-triggered increase in manpower funds praised by Levitan as possibly the most innovative feature proposed by the administration looks relatively trivial. Indeed, although any increase in federal spending triggered automatically by a cyclical downturn fits well with the prejudices of an economist, it is not clear that this increase is particularly well-conceived. If the manpower spending increase because of a rise in unemployment takes the form of higher spending for *training* programs, as indicated in the past by Budget Director Robert Mayo, then the spending might even be counterproductive. To increase training when jobs are becoming less available comes close to nonsense. One major difficulty with many training programs in the past is that trainees were graduated into a declining labor market in which they could make no use of their newly acquired skills; if this is what is proposed again, then we ought to be very wary of the expenditure. If, however, what is being proposed is new *job creation* by the federal government, automatically triggered by an increase in unemployment (the job creation possibly taking place under a subterfuge of training), then it looks like a very good idea indeed. But the direction—training or job creation—is simply not clear. That it should not be just training when unemployment rises is a lesson we should have learned.

Program Unification for Whose Benefit?

Dr. Levitan endorses attempts by the administration and others to pull together all manpower programs under a single legislative authority and a single administrative agency. This is an old disagreement between us.[1] Sar Levitan is accurate in his accusation of overlapping authorities, program duplication, and the like in current manpower programs. From a strictly bureaucratic point of view, it is important to eliminate these; the greatest desideratum of the bureaucratic ethos is to cut off loose threads and to polish up any lack of neatness.

From the viewpoint of program effectiveness in achieving objectives, however, things look quite different. Getting manpower programs properly set up to reach disadvantaged clienteles is a political process as much as a bureaucratic one. It is a political process in which, before 1965, the relevant political forces were the various federal manpower agencies in the Labor Department, the state employment services, and the constituencies of all of these—largely employers and relatively skilled employees using the employment services. The ideology of the agencies was based on the need to run a smooth public employment service, and to do this it was necessary for the service to be responsive to employer needs; otherwise, employers might go elsewhere. But this ideology practically precluded major services to the unskilled workers most in need, because these people were difficult to make attractive to employers.

With the onset of the War on Poverty in 1964, the aim of directing manpower services toward the hard core and other unskilled poor necessitated shaking up the ideology of the manpower agencies, together with a countervailing thrust to oppose the anti-change pressures of the existing manpower constituencies. The Office of Economic Opportunity (OEO) did this initially by setting up rival programs. These programs were intended to act as TVA-type yardsticks, as challenges to the practices of the old manpower bureaucracies, and as competitors. (It has never been clear to me why competition, which is generally rightfully credited with producing better washing machines, should be considered dangerous in any attempt to produce better public programs.)

The challenge and competition to the federal Labor Department came from OEO, the challenge to local manpower bureaucracies from local community action authorities. This early rivalry and its later version—the attempt to set up Concentrated Employment Programs through a sort of competitive cooperation at the national and local levels—worked very well in the objective of redirecting manpower programs toward the poor. These rival programs worked well to this end by the public testimony of the Secretary of Labor, Willard Wirtz; they worked well by the private report of a task force headed by George Shultz, who has of course since replaced Wirtz.

Bureaucratic Change Through Competitive Innovation

In their working, the challenges to the old bureaucracies led to overlap and duplication and all the other bureaucratic sins. And they made the old bureaucracies very uncomfortable. But the manpower bureaucracies did begin to change. They are not fully changed yet, however; it would still be far too easy to consolidate manpower programs under the Manpower Administration and let the old personnel go back to their comfortable ways. This is a likely result of the administration consolidation proposal, and it is particularly likely because of the added fillip in the program, which would move much of the real decision power to the states. "Partnership" between federal and state authorities is a lovely concept, but it is defined programmatically, and in this proposal, the program would put much of the power in the hands of state employment service bureaucracies. And in many states—not all, but many—these bureaucracies are still very unprogressive relative even to national bureaucracies. The proposed manpower consolidation would put training and job programs into a system similar to that by which Title I of the Elementary and Secondary Education Act has been handled by state educational bureaucracies under the general suzerainty of the federal Office of Education, the suzerainty being about as effective as that of the Holy Emperor in the late eighteenth century. If effectiveness in aiding those in need is a primary criterion, Title I has worked badly, and so—it seems likely—will the manpower consolidation proposal. True, the proposed program will result in relatively less duplication and overlap, than at present, but this simply should not be the primary criterion—a familiar disagreement between Sar Levitan and myself.

I also disagree with Sar Levitan's statement in some other less important matters: for example, although I agree with him that JOBS has been oversold, I have some feeling that it is now being underestimated, by him and by others. With all its faults, it is a training and job creation program directed to the poor on a much larger scale than anything which had gone before.

I find myself in major agreement with, and have only praise for, Sar Levitan's usual high standard of precision and factual analysis, by which his statement is a major contribution—in spite of its failure to perceive the light and truth on some important issues—and I only wish his precision were not accompanied by a manpower economist's ethos.

Notes

1. See, for example, Robert Levine, *The Poor Ye Need Not Have With You: Lessons From the War on Poverty* (Cambridge: MIT Press, 1970), pp. 249-50.

Comment

Lisle C. Carter, Jr.

We can all find defects, as well as some valuable things, in the ideas that have been put forth, but what is important, it seems to me, in a program like JOBS, to the extent it is under way, is not so much the specific program itself but the impulses, implicit and expressed, which the program represents.

The Continued Dread of High Unemployment

Despite all the good work that has been done by the Labor Department, the OEO and others, we still are confronted with the rather grim possibility that the unemployment rates for those at the bottom of the labor force are likely to rise to several times the unemployment rate in the labor force in general in the next decade if everything were just to continue as it is. Instead of its running around the current 2:1 ratio, we might anticipate it could run as high as 5:1, or so.

The issue now is, what are we going to do to head off this kind of possibility? It certainly means clearly that we've got to increase the availability of jobs to people at the bottom more rapidly than the economy is growing, and we've got to increase the rate at which they move into those jobs.

To say, as Dr. Levitan does, that existing programs have to go on is to state the obvious; but I think it is legitimately open to question whether these programs are going to be sufficient, whether we can get there from here—that is, can we bring about a closer relation between unemployment rates among nonwhites and the general unemployment rate that we now have. So the issue is not whether these programs are doing some good. The issue is whether they're going to be sufficiently effective and would be sufficiently effective if funded at high levels to change the prospects if one did not intervene substantially in any other way.

If you ask that question, there are at least three kinds of obstacles. One is, not so much the difficulty in the individual who is at the lower end of the labor force, but the difficulties on the side of the employer: the fact that right now employers in general do not see these people—the low-skilled, poorly educated workers, who are increasingly from the nonwhite population—as candidates for jobs that pay well and that have upward mobility. This, in effect, is a disincentive on the demand side, to invade the economist's prerogative.

The Delivery and Control of Services

The second obstacle that I see is the administrative hang-ups in getting manpower services to people in sufficinet quantity to really make any serious impact on the problem that we're dealing with.

The third is the prospect of greater control and manipulation by the purveyors of these services at the local end.

These are obstacles which all of the new or proposed programs are in one way or another addressing. And it seems to me that whether these programs are the answer or not is not really the issue. The issue is whether we recognize these as three serious problems in our current manpower efforts and whether we're going to try to do something about them. I would submit that that is almost basic to breaking out of the rather low level of effectiveness in terms of the overall problem that we have in the manpower field.

The Hard-Core Unemployed and the Subemployed

The disincentive is obvious in low-prestige jobs with poor working conditions, no future, and low pay. Everybody has had the experience of encountering young men who say, "I can stand on the corner and hustle more than you're talking about here." And it's not simply a question of money, it's the interaction between three things: money, the possibility of promotion, and some feeling of autonomy or control over one's own destiny. They'll trade off one for the other, but when you tell them you want them to go into a job that doesn't meet any of those three criteria, then they say, "To hell with you."

I think this problem is an endemic one in the ghetto, and it's endemic not because of the hard-core unemployed, who are really rather the small end of the problem. Anybody who knows how the Johnson Administration got into the problem of hard-core unemployed recognizes it as primarily a political decision. Subemployment figures are much too large to solve by talking about dealing with the problem principally by "getting business into the act," so you say that we have to take a manageable figure. Somebody inevitably says that the hard-core unemployed are 500,000, so let that be our target because that's a manageable number, and let's not talk about millions of people who are subemployed. But from the point of view of people living in the ghetto, the subemployment problem is the reality they perceive every day.

It's the reality not just in economic terms—obviously they're not getting enough money to support families, etc.—but in terms of expectations on the part of the young. Why should they go into employment programs? Why should they stay in school when they have the realistic perception that it really makes no difference whether they graduate from high school or not? They perceive that as a reality, and so this is a real disincentive and we've got to find ways to break that open.

That's why I like to refer to what I have come to call "the virtues of creaming." It seems to me that what is even more important than worrying about the hard-core unemployed at the bottom is trying to move the people who have stable attachment to the labor force up as rapidly as possible—trying to get employers not to look at ghetto residents as a monolith but to see that there are people who are working every day and still can't make enough money to support their families, that there are people who are chronically in and out of jobs because of unsatisfactory experience in whom, presumably, you could develop a greater attachment if they had greater prospects of success.

It seems to me concentration on that end of the problem rather than on the hard-core unemployed would have a multiplier effect as far as the attitude of the young toward many of our manpower and education efforts.

The Problem of Coordination

Then there are the administrative hang-ups. I have struggled with the problem of trying to coordinate things. I think it is a waste of time to talk about coordinating programs as a major way of doing anything about the serious problems that affect large numbers of people. It's not that we don't want to improve our administrative procedures, but one of the things I have found most disappointing about the position paper put out by the National Manpower Policy Task Force was the bland assumption in that paper that if you get public administrative neatness into the program, you're going to have a sizable effect on the outcome of what happens to people in the ghettos. I just think there is no evidence to support that, and it's just absolutely incredible to me that we would take that kind of position.

The assumption that you are going to get a whole range of services and deliver them to people has at least three problems. Are the services in fact available or are we just talking about paper services? There is a real problem of finding resources to provide quality services, and this is one of the reasons, I think, that voluntarism comes in as an effort to patch up that inadequacy.

Another problem is: Do we really know how to coordinate services? And there is little evidence that we do.

The third is: Do services do any good in the end even when we do know how to coordinate them, have the resources and can deliver them? And there is precious little evidence that they do any good.

Welfare Colonialism

And, finally, there is the issue of welfare colonialism, which I think cannot be overlooked. At least when the Community Action agencies were running the manpower programs at the local level, one could have the notion (and I think it might only be a notion) that these programs belonged to the community.

But when you assign (as the Manpower Policy Task Force and, I assume, Secretary Shultz would) all responsibilities to the Employment Service, then there can't be any notion at all that these agencies belong to the people. If the CAA's were being criticized as being too manipulative and too much in control and not giving people enough of a role, what will be said when the Employment Service takes over, particularly when you tie it in more closely with welfare? You are now going to purvey welfare-type services through the Employment Service; that is what you are doing with the notion of offering an array of services. When you tie it with the compulsive aspects of the WIN program, it is perfectly clear that what you have here is just another example of welfare colonialism.

I'm trying to say to you, then, that any response has got to deal with the way people in the ghettos actually feel, young and older people, about programs where they have to go down to "the man" and the man is going to tell them what to do and tell them that if they don't do this, then they don't get that. There has to be a different approach. To the extent that the tax incentive cuts out that middleman or cuts down the middleman relationship and makes it much more a simple referral service but I'm not saying it will necessarily work. I'm saying that that's the kind of problem we have to address.

Continued Experimentation

I am interested in seeing us experiment in other ways. One, which evolved out of a proposal by Robert Levine, is really sort of an individual-benefits system, like a G. I. Bill of Rights for these young people, so they can get the kind of training and offer the kind of incentive to employers that might induce a better bargaining relation at that low end of the labor market.

This would have a lot of wastage in it, just as there was a lot of wastage in the G. I. Bill of Rights, which gave so many people a take-off point. But nobody says now that that program, wastage and all, was not of great benefit to society in the long run, whatever the cost may have been; and nobody at that time was concerned about evaluation and cost-benefit analysis, so we never did know the cost—but I am sure it was astronomical.

Income Maintenance

I would conclude by taking note of income maintenance and its role with respect to manpower programs. We have a kind of discontinuity between the demand for jobs, on the one hand, and the supply, on the other, and we have great difficulty in closing that gap, yet we are faced at the same time with a situation, in urban areas, for example, where 53 per cent of the people are in families who are either working full time or are certainly employable. This is a problem much bigger than that of residual population that can't be expected to make enough money to support itself. Programs to meet the present urgent economic needs of poor workers and at the same time give some stability to that lower end of the labor force while we're trying to work out, through all these experiments, a way to close this gap are of the essence. To state this is to make the case for a *substantial* income-maintenance program as a necessary component, rather than a mere residual, of our approach to solving the nation's manpower problem.

Part 4   Epilogue

8 Toward a Convergence of Economic and Social Policies

George F. Rohrlich

Looking ahead as we enter the 1970's, Professor Hansen has sketched out in his Foreword their probable general economic climate and some problems of public policy pertaining to what he has called "economic mechanics." The editor has attempted to identify certain gaps in the conventional approaches to the study of economics, as well as a number of present-day challenges that bid us transcend some of these past limitations—largely self-imposed—so as to be able to do justice to the pressing socioeconomic issues that demand solutions. The contributing authors and their critics have described in considerable detail the specific problems that pose themselves in three well-defined policy realms: that of social welfare (or social security, in the broad meaning of the term), health care, and manpower and skill development; and they have reviewed and evaluated present and possible alternative approaches in each of these areas.

Meanwhile, reform proposals by the Government that bear on some of these subject matters have undergone preliminary legislative screening and are awaiting consideration by the Congress. The Administration's proposed Manpower Act and its Welfare (Social Security Act) Amendments are particularly relevant. While they touch on matters of health care only peripherally, their combined impact on social welfare—in stepping up work training and employment policies for the nation at large and for the welfare population in particular and in furnishing minimum-income guaranties to an important sector of the working poor not now receiving public support, as well as to welfare recipients—opens up important new dimensions that call for an appraisal. This last chapter constitutes an attempt, necessarily preliminary and aphoristic, to review the draft legislation in historical perspective, with a veiw to identifying the elements of continuity and innovation that it contains, and to appraise the latter in terms of the goals to be achieved.

The Government's Manpower-Reform Plan

The declared purpose of the Manpower Training Act (MTA), the Administration's main instrument for the proposed manpower reforms, is to establish a comprehensive development program "to assist persons in overcoming obstacles to suitable employment," and to "assure meaningful employment opportunities" for workers by enabling them to develop their skills and to realize their full potential.[1] Overall responsibility for the implementation of the Act rests with the Secretary of Labor.

The means envisioned to accomplish the purposes of the Manpower Act are threefold:

1. To augment entry-level opportunities for the placement in private employment of unemployed, underemployed, and low-income workers by assisting those now in entry-level jobs to improve their skills and advance toward more demanding employment;

2. To expand opportunities for such persons to find employment in public-service jobs designed to promote human betterment and public improvement;

3. To provide remedial services to individuals where effective opportunities have not been provided or access to them continues to be restricted, including specifically opportunities for training, placing and upgrading public assistance recipients with a view to developing their capacity for self-support.[2]

By restructuring, consolidation, administrative and financial revamping of present manpower programs, it is intended to create an integrated and comprehensive manpower service system for the nation involving all sectors of the economy and all levels of government. By means of this system, "employability development plans" are to be designed to fit individual needs for any persons whose participation in such a program could be expected to improve the utilization of the nation's manpower resources.

Remuneration and cash supports for the participants in any facet of this program should create or reenforce incentives to undergo training and establish rewards for its successful completion. Base pay for all trainees will equal 40 per cent of average wages paid in employments covered by the state's unemployment compensation law (rising gradually to 50 per cent from the third year of operations) plus $5 per week for each dependent, up to and including the sixth. A completion bonus of twice the weekly amounts would be given those completing authorized training courses and 15 weeks' duration or longer.

Recipients of welfare payments would continue to receive these while undergoing training and, in addition, would be paid a monthly expense allowance of $30 for each member of a participating family (or more, if training allowances for a family under another program exceeded this combination by more than $30 per member) plus compensation for travel and other extra costs.

Workers employed in "work-experience" programs will be paid wages at rates at least equivalent to the minimum prescribed by the Fair Labor Standards Act (FLSA). Those undergoing on-the-job training in private employment will be paid at this same rate or at the locally prevailing wage rate if it is higher than the FLSA minimum. This applies without distinction as to age to those of legal working age 16 and up.

Incentives are built also into the proposed financing of programs under the MTA. These incentives are aimed at three different objectives: (1) coordinating with nationally set priorities, but at the same time decentralizing to state and local levels, the planning and delivery of manpower services; (2) rewarding excellence in performance and financial initiative at local levels; (3) stimulating additional training activities when the economy is sagging.

The first objective, coordination and decentralization of planning, is to be achieved in successive stages whereby states will obtain direct authority over 25 per cent and 66-2/3 per cent, respectively, of the total allocation to them of MTA moneys (aggregating 75 per cent of the total federal appropriations, apportioned among the states in amounts that reflect labor-force participation, unemployment, and poverty in each state as compared with the national average). To achieve stage one, a state must devise a comprehensive plan that is in conformity with the overall (national) plan and embraces at least the services provided under the MTA and those provided by the Employment Service, under the financial administration of a single state agency designated by the Governor. To achieve the second stage, the state plan must comprise all manpower and related activities and must operate under a state comprehensive manpower agency, with prime sponsors, designated by the Governor (and aided by area advisory bodies), in each major metropolitan area.

The second objective, to reward excellence and financial initiative, will be furthered by rewarding states with 100 per cent administration of MTA-granted funds when state-local partnership meets exemplary standards of performance, to be established by the Secretary; and by federal matching in a ratio of 2:1 of any additional state funds committed to manpower programs. (Five per cent of the Federal MTA appropriation, in addition to the 75 per cent referred to above, is earmarked for this purpose.)

The third objective, a counter-recessionary set-up of training, is to be served by an automatic increase in MTA moneys whenever the ratio of unemployment has attained or exceeded 4.5 per cent for any consecutive three-month period. A complementary provision is to take effect at a somewhat later point: the automatic extension by an extra 13 weeks of the maximum period of compensable unemployment whenever the rate of insured unemployment for the nation as a whole has attained or exceeded 4.5 per cent (equal to about 6 per cent of that total unemployment) for any consecutive three-month period. This is not part of the MTA bill but is a provision contained in the pending Employment Security (Unemployment Insurance) Amendments. It is expected to be tied into the former, however, by enabling workers experiencing prolonged unemployment to use the extended compensation to take MTA-authorized training.

Several further tools are to be used to promote expeditious and efficient worker placement. One is the development of job banks, i.e., computerized job-location and job-seeker matching operations (ultimately nationwide). Another is the experimental funneling of job-vacancy information to unemployment insurance claimants directly from the Unemployment Insurance office (by-passing the Employment Service). Yet another is the development of a multiple-track system of Employment Service clients, with a view to separating those with limited service needs from those with extensive service requirements. A fourth pertains to the continuation of relocation assistance for unemployed workers with definite job offers in distant locations. A fifth is the development of an employment security automated reporting system, a tracking device that will serve as an important research tool in that it should furnish a basis for evaluating, through follow-up of the employment and work experience of workers, the effectiveness of the several modes of employment assistance.

The Government's Welfare-Reform Plan

The core of the proposed welfare reforms is the President's "Family Assistance Plan," viewed by him as "a totally new approach to welfare, designed to assist those left far behind the national norm, and provide all with the motivation to work and a fair share of the opportunity to train."[3]

The plan treats the welfare problem, insofar as possible, as a part of the larger problem complex of manpower development, employability, and employment promotion: "We have stopped considering human welfare in isolation. The new plan is part of an overall approach which includes a comprehensive new Manpower Training Act . . ."[4]

The Secretary of Health, Education and Welfare and the Secretary of Labor further stressed this intent in their testimonies, the former by referring to the "supporting work-oriented family assistance program" as the last in a threesome with "the emphasis . . . first and principally on jobs, second on an assured income growing out of social security [social insurance] . . ." The latter by making the point that "*work* is a major feature of this program." Thus representing the President's Family Assistance Plan (FAP) as "a program of support for those who demonstrate a willingness to help themselves," they went so far as to state that it was "not an income guarantee . . . *not a* proposal for a guaranteed minimum income."[5] This assertion, though inaccurate if taken literally, was meant to bring out, no doubt, the distinction between a "guaranteed minimum income (GMI) *for everyone*" (emphasis supplied), which the President had discarded as one of several undesirable alternatives to the course actually chosen.

The provisions for payment of Family Assistance Benefits (FAB) by the Secretary of Health, Education and Welfare are intended to replace those now providing for grants to states for Aid and Services to Needy Families with Children (AFDC). Eligible for FAB will be families with children (below age 18, or 21 if regularly attending school) as long as family income (other than that which is excluded in the computation) and the family's resources (other than their home, household goods, personal effects and other property essential to the family's self-support) do not exceed stated limits. Benefits will be paid at the rate of $500 per year for each of the first two (related) members and $300 for each additional member. If the family has other income, it may keep in any one year the first $720 of earned family income plus 50 per cent of the remainder (with certain exceptions) and also 50 per cent of unearned income (with stated exceptions).[6] The income of a family of four would range from $1,600 to $3,920 per year, plus food stamps, which would raise the range to $2,350-$4,000.

In principle, adult able-bodied recipients of FAB who are of working age and are not in full-time employment must register for manpower services, training or employment; those disabled are to be referred for rehabilitation. Such registration is optional for mothers of children under six and for specified others who take care of children or of household members who are sick. In all other cases, failure to register leads to forfeiture of that individual's (not the family's) FAB.

Whenever benefits fall below those formerly payable under the AFDC program, the state must supplement FAB up to that amount (except in case of the working poor) and allow retention of earnings at prescribed rates, failing which the state forfeits federal subsidies for other federal-state public-assistance programs. Conversely, additional federal subsidies will assure that the state's total costs are kept at no more than 90 per cent of what they would be in the absence of the FAP amendments.

Several significant innovations apply to the three categorical programs—Aid to the Aged (AA), Aid to the Blind (AB), and Aid to the Permanently and Totally Disabled (APTD)—which, unlike AFDC, will continue essentially as now operating. One is the provision of a minimum monthly benefit of $90, with the proviso that states paying more now must not lower their benefit amounts. This stipulation would be a federal requirement and would take the place of current provisions, stating merely that state standards for determining eligibility and amount of aid must be reasonable. Income from other sources, and resources that can be disregarded in certifying need at this minimum amount, are to be defined more uniformly and more broadly than at present, as they are under the FAP.

The most important aspect of the proposed FAP and the changes in the three remaining categorical assistance programs is the assurance of a guaranteed minimum income for all persons comprised thereunder (i.e., the nearly 10 million persons on welfare and the estimated 10 million working poor, with their families) except any individuals subject to the requirement of work or work training conceivably failing to comply with this requirement for reasons not deemed justified.

With regard to the delivery of manpower-training and related services to FAB recipients, the Administration's manpower reforms become directly applicable to the welfare reforms. The tie-in is accomplished by virtue of a section of the Manpower Training Act which is intended to replace in its entirety that part of the Social Security Act containing the work-incentive (WIN) provisions, built into the AFDC program by the 1967 Welfare Amendments. While various laws and their differential financing provisions are involved in the effectuation of the aforementioned measures, those under MTA and specifically those affecting FAB recipients would be underwritten at (or up to) a rate of 90 per cent from the federal MTA appropriations to the Secretary of Labor. Insofar as the policies and programs affect FAB recipients, the concurrence of the Secretary of Health, Education and Welfare (HEW) will be required with respect to those traditionally under the authority of that department.

In order to make training programs and gainful employment in fact accessible to mothers of young children, the Welfare Reform Act stipulates that the Secretary of Health, Education and Welfare "shall make provision for the furnishing of child care services in such cases and for so long as he deems appropriate in the case of individuals registered . . . who are . . . participating in manpower services, training or employment." To this effect, the Secretary is authorized to pay up to 90 per cent of the cost of projects for child care and related services for persons so registered and participating; and the remaining 10 per cent (the nonfederal share of the cost) may take the form of services or facilities.[7]

The Background of Social Welfare Legislation

By virtue of the fact that the reforms extend the national concern for manpower development to a target population which overlaps the welfare clientele (some part-time and irregular members and some that are merely potential members of the labor force) and which includes others (the working poor) who are a proper concern for social policy, and also by virtue of the extensive use of the cash-subsidization method, which has long been the mainstay of public assistance, they mark a high point in the convergence of manpower and welfare policies that has been in the making for some time.

Our concern with social welfare is the older of the two, and a national commitment in this area came about earlier than in that of manpower development. The start of the modern era in social-welfare thinking in the United States may be pinpointed fairly accurately—at least as far as concrete results in the shape of legislation and operating programs are concerned—to the 1930's, specifically the Social Security Act of 1935. What had gone before, in the wake of the economic crash and the Depression, was sheer makeshift and experimentation—imaginative and bold, to be sure, but improvised for the sake of momentary relief and, perhaps even more, to show that there were things we could do to ban the fear which, according to President Franklin Delano Roosevelt's famous words, was the only thing to be feared.

The Social Security Act went far beyond all that. It was truly a new departure, the start on a long road or, as President Roosevelt remarked in signing the Act, "a cornerstone in a structure that was being built" and which, though "far from complete" had a distinct philosophy and clear-cut objective. The philosophy was to provide for the essentials in an orderly, planful and dignified fashion, so that people—all people—no longer able to do so by their own efforts or with their family's support, could confront the common contingencies of life with confidence. The objective was to achieve this within a federal-state setting in a gradualist manner, i.e., by developing and expanding the system's protective fabric so as to give it broader scope and depth of cover, as and when called for and deemed feasible. The unemployed, the old, and fatherless children were the first to obtain consideration and a measure of relief; social hazards not initially covered were to be provided for in due time, and other groups in need of protection were to be added. Presumptive need or actual need, depending on the type of program, was to govern benefit determination, and most important of all, social security benefits were to be paid as of right.

The right-to-benefit concept became firmly entrenched, both in program design and in people's awareness, in at least one type of social security program, the social insurances. Their contributory character readily lent to the benefits awarded the earmarks of an earned right. It was by no means absent, however, from the categorical public-assistance programs. The many guaranties aimed at their universal availability within the state, their impartial and efficient administration, and the equitable adjudication of benefits that were written into the several assistance titles of the Social Security Act give proof of that.

The weakness of the concept, when applied to the federally subsidized assistance programs, was not to be found in the fact that, by definition, entitlement under each of these was conditional upon a test of need and, consequently, of the means of the persons to be aided. Rather, it was a double uncertainty built into the law. First and foremost, the proviso "as far as practicable under the conditions of such State, to furnish financial assistance,"[8] which is part of the appropriation (federal-state matching) provisions of the Social Security Act, left the extent and adequacy of funding relative to need uncertain. Secondly, and at least in part a consequence of this downward-pointed open-endedness, the absence of statutory minimum levels of assistance and measures of need precluded any assurance of implementation pursuant to advance specifications. Administrative standards and regulatory procedures could ameliorate but never remedy this twin defect, for the simple reason that lack of state funding could effectively undercut them. In recent years, nevertheless, both nationally and in an increasing number of states, the right-to-benefit issue has been revived and the concept has gained ground, as well as some practical implementation. Cases in point are the ruling by the Supreme Court of the United States declaring state residence requirements unconstitutional; the discard of the man-in-the-house search; and most recently, the Supreme Court ruling requiring notice and hearing before termination of benefit payment. These developments have been favored by a general climate of good will toward the disadvantaged, a widespread desire to help Negroes in their quest for de facto emancipation, the pressure of some self-help organizations, and a surging interest in welfare law and in the social-welfare aspects of the law in general.

Comparable far-reaching goals in the field of employment and manpower were raised by the Committee on Economic Security, which in 1934-35 did all the preparatory work for the development and formulation of the social security program. In fact, the very first item in the Committee's *Report to the President* called for an "Employment Assurance" as the necessary premise for other Committee recommendations, notably a program of unemployment insurance.[9] However, this issue was raised only to be forgotten for many years and, to date, it has not entered into any federal or state statute or program. What ensued instead, under the "Employment Security" label (and what has remained for most of the intervening years), was the combined job-placement and unemployment-compensation functions based on the Wagner-Peyser and Social Security Acts, and the corresponding state laws that implemented the program's intent and financed provisions of those federal statutes. In a somewhat similar vein, the call for federal legislation to assure full employment raised in the wake of the extraordinary and highly successful manpower efforts made during World War II, merely led to the Employment Act of 1946, which declared reasonably full employment to be one of several policy concerns of the federal government.

On the sidelines, a continuing and very slowly increasing interest in vocational rehabilitation for the disabled was kept alive by the then Office of

Vocational Rehabilitation (OVR). It received something of a boost in connection with the establishment of the categorical public-assistance program of Aid to the Permanently and Totally Disabled (APTD) and more thereafter, in connection with the advent of disability insurance in the early 1950's and its expansion in the mid-1950's. In fact, the OVR was probably the first federal agency that tried to base its case as much as possible on the investment-in-man concept and on the persuasiveness of certain limited cost-benefit analyses.

A more widespread interest in manpower matters was aroused by various studies and reports on northern and western European (notably the Swedish and the European Economic Community) programs for manpower development through skill training and worker mobility. To unfreeze some of the ample and—from a socioeconomic point of view almost completely sterile—unemployment insurance reserves for similar purposes was a slow, uphill struggle.

Thus, it was not until the lingering and slowly rising unemployment levels of the late 1950's and early 1960's began seriously to worry us and the issue of structural unemployment, thought to be resistant to absorption by stepped-up aggregate demand, attracted attention in its own right that one could speak of the beginning of a positive or active manpower program. It began with the adoption of the Area Redevelopment legislation in 1961 (to cope with the "pockets of poverty," the common euphemism at the time), which was followed, in short succession, by the Manpower Development and Training Act in 1962 and the Economic Opportunity Act in 1964. Sandwiched in between was the first "live" and the most interesting large-scale demonstration project in remedial education, training and employment promotion for young people: Mobilization for Youth, in New York City.

The growing number of welfare recipients could not escape attention in this connection. The program of Aid to Dependent Children (ADC) became one of Aid and Services to Needy Families with Children (AFDC), what with a growing awareness, first of all, that its early program design had done nothing to change—except possibly for the worse—a situation where such child dependency was accompanied by the forced absence from the house of an unemployed or underemployed father; and second, that possibilities for rehabilitiation of adult beneficiaries of the program and, more important, of families, were not being tested in any systematic manner. President Kennedy reflected the new mood of Congress and the Administration in the early 1960's when he advocated "stressing services instead of support, rehabilitation instead of relief, and training for useful work instead of prolonged dependency."[10]

The 1962 Welfare Amendments to the Social Security Act brought the first major reform along these lines. Evaluations of their effectiveness based on experience have not been numerous or conclusive. However, clear testimony of Congress's adverse judgment on their effectiveness is available in the form of the 1967 Welfare Amendments. Frequently interpreted as an expression of Congress's alleged resolve to "get tough," which may be as difficult to prove as to gainsay, they reveal incontestably a three-pronged attack on the further growth of this particular welfare program. One of the three curbs (the imposition of limits on case loads) was first postponed and later abandoned. The two remaining make up the current Work Incentive (WIN) program. They constitute a drastic application of the new manpower preoccupation: (1) to maximize labor force participation through promoting training and gainful employment opportunities; and (2) to remove any work disincentives that might hamper this reorientation. The "tough" requirement of mandated work for welfare mothers, which aroused much indignation, was attenuated in practice by the nonavailability of day-care centers to look after their children—this being both a practical and a statutory condition for the enforcement of the work-or-training mandate. In fact, therefore, the concomitant commitment to provide more such facilities may be viewed mainly as a pledge to remove yet another disincentive.

This is where we stood when the Nixon Administration's proposals for manpower and welfare reforms were being advanced. The reforms have been represented as an altogether new approach to social welfare. Viewed in historical perspective, however, they combine the partial fulfillment of a long-standing commitment in welfare policy proper (the right to benefit) with greater emphasis on another standing commitment (child care and support). Their most innovative feature is the extension of manpower policies by the application of methods not previously tried (wage subsidies) to problem areas (marginal employment and earnings) that have eluded successful intervention by other means. In terms of motivation, a desire for the fullest possible application of manpower training and employment promotion measures to all sectors of the actual and potential labor force in the interest of full employment and economic growth would appear to have a stronger claim to godfathership of the present reforms than our older, but as yet not nearly so effective, concern for social policy.

Harnessing Program Design to Policy Objectives

On the whole, then, the reforms may fairly be interpreted as a concerted effort to reaffirm and partly restate established public policies with regard to employment and manpower, on the one hand, and with regard to social security, i.e., its bottom layer, public assistance or public welfare (in a narrow sense), on the other. A trend toward a limited convergence between these two policy areas, clearly in evidence prior to the present reforms, is being reinforced and stepped up. Viewed from the manpower side, the training component of an invigorated and streamlined positive manpower policy is to be pushed to new lengths by extending the gamut of manpower services, oriented toward gainful employment, to the welfare population and to the working poor, along with all other sectors of the population that might benefit from them. Viewed from the welfare side, the statutory assurance of specified benefit amounts as of right to those meeting stated conditions of eligibility is being extended beyond the social insurance sector into the programs of last resort to ward off dependence. The concept and system of social security as an undertaking by government to provide through a network of programs or provisions for basic protection in common contingencies *as of right,* is thus being implemented more fully than heretofore.

The issues of work and income from transfer payments are joined in the work test administered to all recipients of welfare payments who are presumed to be capable of and available for work or work training, i.e., all except those excused by reason of old age, disability, or illness or because they are in charge of young children. For those subject to the work test, the terms of payment of the transfer income are assimilated to those governing the pay of other trainees, on-the-job learners, and workers generally, i.e., trainees or workers who drop out forfeit their pay. In the case of the welfare recipients under reference, this is construed to mean their own (but not their dependents') portion of the transfer payment. Thus, the sanction constitutes a proviso, or condition—viz., the acceptance and continued pursuit of work and training opportunities—to the continued receipt of the transfer payment by those not previously eligible to such a payment at all, i.e., able-bodied persons below age 65 other than AFDC mothers. There is no change in the letter of the law as regards AFDC mothers with children above age 6; for under the present WIN program they (and, at present, mothers with younger children, too) are required to accept work or training. Whether or not it will de facto constitute a change—in that a provision largely unenforced at present might have teeth put into it—remains to be seen. The de facto proviso applying in the form of lack of day-care centers seems likely to continue for some time. For the present, it seems proper to conclude that the conditions governing eligibility for and continued receipt of the newly added transfer payments for able-bodied persons of working age are those normally governing earned income. With regard to this group of FAB recipients, then, welfare policy has been merged with manpower (work-training and employment) policy.

From the vantage point of a holistic, i.e., comprehensive and consistent, social policy position, how do the reforms measure up to ultimate objectives?

The success of work-training and other forms of upgrading a worker's usable skills and earning capacity must be judged, ultimately, by the test of suitable job placement. This presupposes more or better employment opportunities in the private or the public sector or in both. The reforms make reference to this ultimate goal but do not make clear how the hoped-for numerical and qualitative improvement in job opportunities is to come about. Especially with regard to youth unemployment, the absence of any assured employment—if necessary, by the government as employer of last resort—would appear to leave a meticulously thought out job-preparatory program without the necessary safeguards for its intended consummation. Even the counter-recessionary automatic increase in Manpower Training Act appropriations will serve to augment merely the training opportunities, not necessarily the job openings. This could aggravate rather than help an existing problem situation. Since for the overwhelming majority of Americans, uninterrupted gainful employment will offer the only assurance of a continuing flow of income in the foreseeable future, the only ultimate guaranty of this is an employment assurance of the type demanded 35 years ago by the Committee on Economic Security. Despite the present emphasis on work and gainful employment, this is not a part of the proposed work-income provisions. In fact, the Secretary of Labor pronounced himself decidedly in opposition to this idea.[11]

Short of employment guaranties, the maximization of job placement must rest on incentives. This, indeed, is the tool or vehicle favored in the present reforms. Presumably, the differential, regular, and incentive pay provisions applying to trainees, on-the-job learners, and FAB recipients, respectively, are intended to provide adequate incentives to the job seekers. The absence of special pay scales applicable to young persons of working age, on the other hand, would appear to pass up the opportunity to provide an incentive to employers to hire teenagers in larger numbers. With youth (teen-age) unemployment long the heaviest and most vexing of all unemployment, the attempt to step up on-the-job training and employment of youngsters by private employers through the institution of youth wages below the general minimum established by the Federal Labor Standards Act seems worth trying. Such differential minimum-wage provisions, quite common abroad, might be one means of neutralizing existing employer disincentives to hire youths, such as the military draft, restrictions concerning types and hours of work, etc.[12] Whether by this or other means, the problem of massive youth unemployment clearly calls for higher priority attention than is accorded it in the reforms, both for its own sake, and by reason of its leverage in solving the social-problem syndrome of the urban slum.

How will those fare under the new scheme of things who are without a job and in need or, for that matter, with a job but still in need? Here the welfare reform will have a threefold impact. Those aged, blind, or otherwise totally and permanently disabled and in need are assured of receiving public assistance—some in more ample amounts than at present, owing to the new federal minimum-benefit standard; and some for the first time, owing to the streamlined and liberalized eligibility rules. The coutinued need and justification for this type of cash subsidy are beyond question or controversy. What it leaves unanswered is the plight of a person in need (conceivably even after training) who is neither old nor totally and permanently disabled. Unless such a person has charge of a dependent child, he or she must continue to depend on the fortuities of general relief, provided in very limited and often haphazard ways by state and local governments, and on private charity. Despite proven need and attested failure to obtain gainful employment, even after training, such persons will continue to be, as they are now, without any entitlement to public aid. In a program that purports to mesh maximum efforts at work training and employment with "proper care for the dependent" whose needs are not susceptible to being met in this way, this failure to afford some last-line across-the-board protection defies the President's test, according to which "A measure of the greatness of a powerful nation is the character of the life it creates for those who are powerless to make ends meet."[13]

The two other points of impact of the new legislation affect families (including broken families) with dependent children and in need through what, in effect, amounts to (1) a family allowance, supplemented in some cases by (2) a low-earnings or employment subsidy. These are new types of cash subsidization. Both are amply justified and needed from a social-policy standpoint. The latter because—if employment is to be maximized—some submarginal employment, and for some time probably a considerable amount of it, will have to be part of the total employment effort. However, in light of this policy objective, it is hard to find a plausible explanation for the exclusion from such subsidized employment opportunities of single workers without dependent children and, most of all, of working-age youngsters. A different, less disguised form of low-earnings or employment subsidy, more broadly conceived, might better meet the policy goal.

Regarding the family allowance component of the FAP, a clarification of the purpose it can and should serve within a broad and coherent policy framework, likewise, might suggest a rather different program design. What justifies a family-oriented social subsidy is, presumably, a public concern with optimum family formation and family maintenance. This concern may be classed, to be sure, under the rubric of policies designed to assure adequate incomes. But in light of its focus on families with children, that program feature, surely, partakes necessarily of another social policy area—the public concern with population. In fact, the specific difference that would seem to warrant the limited focus can hardly be the contingent need for income supports, which, after all, is not circumscribed in this particular manner.

Presumably, it is a public concern with the family as the source of our future population.

If this is a valid interpretation of the inherent rationale of family-and-child focused income supports—whether or not it is explicitly stated to be the objective of the particular program—then the weight of incentives and the distribution in the allocation of any given amount of funds should be such as to enhance progress toward attainment of that primary policy objective. The payment of a rather small subsidy in respect of each and every child born into a family may not constitute an incentive for families to have more children. But payment of a substantial amount in respect of only a limited number of children is likely to offer a significant disincentive to having more.[14] What kind of design would give maximum leverage to a quality-oriented family-benefit program?

Clearly, the twin aim must be to keep the number of children down and to afford them the care they need while young. Consequently, for mothers who stay at home to take care of preschool or school-age children—and only for such mothers—a substantial subsidy to enable her to do so would seem well taken. It is certainly one instance of justified disincentive to work dictated by social-policy considerations. Similarly, there is every reason to pay a substantial subsidy in respect of the first two or at most three children (and only these). In extending these subsidies, there would be no need to make eligibility contingent on the parties' limited income or on property and other restrictive conditions. Rather, the task of wiping out most of the cash subsidy of the upper-income families could be entrusted safely and efficiently to the administration of appropriately restructured tax provisions.

Obviously, all children born into a family (despite any financial disincentive) must be taken care of. This points, once more, to the imperative need for a last line of defense against adversities of whatever source. Such programs exist in a number of countries, notably the United Kingdom, Canada, and other British Commonwealth countries. Commonly called social assistance, they take the form of noncategorical public assistance programs assuring a guaranteed minimum income to all in need, on the basis of a simplified and generalized means test, but as a matter of right. The addition to our social security fabric of such a catch-all last line of defense would complete the realization, at long last, of the right-to-benefit promise inherent in the social security concept adopted in this country as a national policy in 1935. It would provide the minimum-income guaranty for any needy child and for any adult who, despite being of working age and not having a dependent child in his or her custody, either cannot work or, if working, cannot support himself from his earnings. Thus, it would close the work-income and needs gap for all those for whom the present reforms fail to accomplish this.

Notes

1. Manpower Training Act, Preamble and Section 2.

2. Ibid., Section 2, paragraphs 3-6.

3. Committee on Ways and Means, House of Representatives, *The President's Proposals for Welfare Reform,* 91st Cong., 1st sess., October 1969, p. 94.

4. Ibid.

5. Committee on Ways and Means, *Written Statements by Administration Witnesses . . . at Hearings on Social Security and Welfare Proposals,* 91st Cong., 1st sess., October 15, 1969, pp. 1, 24, and 39.

6. The Committee on Ways and Means, in reporting favorably on the bill on March 11, 1970, discarded this 50 per cent retention clause in respect of nonearned income in favor of a dollar-for-dollar offset. See *Family Assistance Act of 1970.* Report of the Committee on Ways and Means on H. R. 16311. Report No. 91-904, 91st Cong., 2nd sess., Washington, Government Printing Office, 1970. Surprisingly, old-age, survivors, and disability insurance benefits, as well as employment benefits, are treated as nonearned, rather than earned, income.

7. Welfare Reform Act, Sections 447-c and 437.

8. See Section 1 of Titles I, IV, X, XIV, XVI of the Social Security Act.

9. Committee on Economics Security, *Report to the President* (Washington, D. C.: U. S. Government Printing Office, 1935), p. 3.

10. Quoted by Leonard J. Hausman in "From Welfare Rolls to Payrolls? The Welfare System as a Manpower and Rehabilitiation System" *Public-Private Manpower Policies,* edited by A. R. Weber, *et al.* (Madison, Wisc.: Industrial Relations Research Association, 1969), pp. 135-136.

11. Committee on Ways and Means, *Written Statements,* p. 64.

12. These issues are discussed by T. W. Gavett in light of a recent Department of Labor survey in "Youth Unemployment and Minimum Wages," *Monthly Labor Review,* March 1970, pp. 3-12.

13. This is the opening sentence in the President's Message on Welfare Reform of August 11, 1969. See *The President's Proposals for Welfare Reform,* p. 93.

14. It is significant, in this context, that in France, the country that pioneered with regard to family-allowance programs and which operates the most substantial programs of this type, a seasoned student of the subject recently made the following observation: "It does seem that family benefits have an appreciable effect on the birth rate, less perhaps by the material contribution they make to families than by the climate that they help create around childbirth and the idea of the family." Pierre Laroque, "Social Security in France," *Social Security in International Perspective,* edited by Shirley Jenkins (New York: Columbia University Press, 1969), p. 182.

About the Editor

George F. Rohrlich is Professor of Political Economy and Social Insurance at the School of Business Administration, Temple University, where he established and now directs the Institute for Social Economics. He holds a J.D. degree from the University of Vienna and a Ph.D. degree from Harvard University and was a Research Training Fellow at the Brookings Institution. Dr. Rohrlich has held research and planning positions in the United States Government and in international administration, primarily in the field of social security. He has taught at Sweet Briar College, the University of Chicago, Columbia University, and the University of Trieste, Italy, and is the author of numerous publications on various aspects of social economics. In 1970 he was appointed a member of the Joint WHO-ILO Committee of Experts on Personal Health Care and Social Security.

Contributors
and Discussants

Eveline M. Burns is Professor at the Graduate School of Social Work, New York University, and Professor Emeritus, Columbia University. She holds a Ph.D. degree from the London School of Economics, of which she is an Honorary Fellow, and honorary doctorates from several American universities. She has held numerous executive and advisory positions in federal and state government agencies and in national and international professional and civic organizations. Dr. Burns has to her credit a long list of publications on social security and social welfare policy.

Robert J. Lampman is Professor of Economics at the University of Wisconsin and is a staff member of the Institute for Research on Poverty and Editor of the *Journal of Human Resources*. He holds a Ph.D. degree from the University of Wisconsin. He has served with the Council of Economic Advisers and as a consultant to other agencies of the federal government. He is the author of several books and many articles, notably in the field of income distribution.

Sar A. Levitan is Research Professor of Economics and Director of the Center for Manpower Policy Studies at George Washington University. He received his Ph.D. degree from Columbia University. He has held various teaching assignments and research and advisory positions in government and nonprofit organizations, and has published extensively, especially on manpower and antipoverty programming and program evaluation.

Garth L. Mangum is McGraw Professor of Economics and Director of the Human Resources Institute at the University of Utah, as well as Research Professor of Economics and Co-Director of the Center for Manpower Policy Studies at George Washington University. He received his Ph.D. degree from Harvard University. He has held various research and executive positions with Congressional and Presidential agencies concerned with national manpower policies and has published widely in this area.

Gerard Piel is a cofounder, President, and Publisher of *Scientific American*. He has an A.B. degree *magna cum laude* from Harvard University and a series of honorary doctor's degrees from American and Canadian universities. A Fellow of the American Academy of Arts and Sciences and of the American Association for the Advancement of Science, he served as Chairman of the Commission on the Delivery of Personal Health Services, New York City (1967-68).

Herman M. Somers is a Professor of Politics and Public Affairs at the Woodrow Wilson School of Princeton University. He holds a Ph.D. degree from Harvard University. In addition to a long career in college and university teaching, he has to his credit service in State and Federal government positions, including several Presidential Task Forces and National Advisory Councils and Committees. He has authored and co-authored several books and numerous articles on health care and social security.

* * * * *

Lisle C. Carter, Jr., is Vice-President for Social and Environmental Studies of Cornell University and a former Assistant Secretary of Health, Education and Welfare.

Henry H. Chase is Coordinator for Social Legislation with the Tax Department of the Humble Oil and Refining Company. He is a member of the Social Security Commission of the Chamber of Commerce of the United States.

Nelson H. Cruikshank is a member of the National Council of Churches' Department on the Church and Economic Life and of the Health Insurance Benefits Advisory Council (on Medicare).

Howard Ennes is Second Vice-President of the Equitable Life Assurance Society of the United States.

William L. Kissick, M.D., is Professor and Chairman of the Department of Community Medicine at the University of Pennsylvania; he has served as Executive Director of the National Advisory Commission on Health Facilities.

Robert A. Levine is associated with the RAND Corporation. He is a former Assistant Director for Research, Plans, Programs and Evaluation of the Office of Economic Opportunity.

Howard Rosen is Director of the Office of Manpower Research, U.S. Department of Labor.

Bert Seidman is Director of the AFL-CIO Social Security Department.

Michael K. Taussig is Professor of Economics at Rutgers–The State University.

Date Due

JUL 9 78